PHILOSOPHY OF MIND

SERIES EDITOR
David J. Chalmers, Australian National University and New York University

The Peripheral Mind

Philosophy of Mind and the
Peripheral Nervous System

István Aranyosi

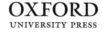
OXFORD
UNIVERSITY PRESS

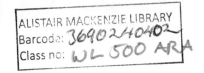

OXFORD
UNIVERSITY PRESS

Oxford University Press is a department of the University of Oxford.
It furthers the University's objective of excellence in research, scholarship,
and education by publishing worldwide.

Oxford   New York
Auckland   Cape Town   Dar es Salaam   Hong Kong   Karachi
Kuala Lumpur   Madrid   Melbourne   Mexico City   Nairobi
New Delhi   Shanghai   Taipei   Toronto

With offices in
Argentina   Austria   Brazil   Chile   Czech Republic   France   Greece
Guatemala   Hungary   Italy   Japan   Poland   Portugal   Singapore
South Korea   Switzerland   Thailand   Turkey   Ukraine   Vietnam

Oxford is a registered trademark of Oxford University Press
in the UK and certain other countries.

Published in the United States of America by
Oxford University Press
198 Madison Avenue, New York, NY 10016

© Oxford University Press 2013

Library of Congress Cataloging-in-Publication Data
Aranyosi, István.
The peripheral mind : philosophy of mind and the peripheral nervous system /
István Aranyosi.
p. cm. — (Philosophy of mind)
Includes bibliographical references and index.
ISBN 978–0–19–998960–7 (hardback : alk. paper) — ISBN 978–0–19–998961–4 (updf)
1. Philosophy of mind.   2. Nerves, Peripheral.   3. Cognition—Philosophy.
4. Externalism (Philosophy of mind)   5. Nervous system–Psychological
aspects.   I. Title.
BD418.3.A73 2013
128'.2–dc23
2012043548

1 3 5 7 9 8 6 4 2
Printed in the United States of America
on acid-free paper

To Ezgi

"Why don't I keep sleeping for a little while longer and forget all this foolishness," he thought. But this was entirely impractical, for he was used to sleeping on his right side…

Franz Kafka, *Metamorphosis*

Contents

Part IV. Mind and Ethics 173

Preface and Acknowledgments

The genesis of this book is unusual as compared to the way the standard monograph in contemporary philosophy comes to see the light of day. I had no fellowship, sabbatical leave, special funding, etc. that I could now acknowledge; the manuscript is not based on any materials that I previously published; I have not presented parts of it at any conference, and, with a few important exceptions, I was too shy to bother colleagues in the field to read it and offer me feedback on it. The important exceptions are Ben Blumson, Weng Hong Tang, and Mike Pelczar from National University of Singapore, who were very kind to have organized a reading group around the manuscript, unfolding over several months, as the manuscript was being written here in Ankara. In November 2011 they invited me to Singapore, where we discussed many problems related to the manuscript. I am grateful to Ben for this visit and for organizing the reading group at his department. I would like to also mention David Chalmers, who read a few of the opening chapters, and, with his proverbial light-speed, promptly offered some very encouraging feedback. His excitement over this project gave me a lot of encouragement and energy to complete the book in a very short time. I'm also grateful to my colleagues from Bilkent University who responded promptly in conversation or writing when there was something I needed feedback on, especially Kourken Michaelian, who made me think more about memory the Extended Mind Hypothesis, Bill Wringe who raised some question related to philosophical theories of perception (a topic that meantime I decided not to include in this book, as

I thought I did not have enough original points to make), and William Coker, who called my attention to Julian Jaynes's work and also checked some parts of the manuscript for style. My brief correspondence with Fabrizio Benedetti and Shaun Gallagher also proved very useful for the discussion of proprioception in chapter 7.

Another unusual feature of the genesis of this book is that it was virtually written "in one breath" and it was not preceded by any planning. As a matter of fact, I had been working for some months on another book, titled *God, Mind, and Logical Space*, when in June 2011, without any warning or explanation, I found myself writing the first pages of what at the time I preferred to be titled *The Marginal Mind*, which then became *The Peripheral Mind* following Dave Chalmers's suggestion. I wrote the book between June and December 2011. This, of course, does not mean that the ideas I am discussing in the book, and especially the main points about the empirical and conceptual role of the Peripheral Nervous System, had not been at the back of my mind for quite some time, only that before actually writing, it had never occurred to me that I could write a book on these issues. Writing it felt very enjoyable, gratifying, and exciting. Most of it was written during the summer break in our holiday house, in a small Turkish town on the shores of the Aegean Sea, Kuşadası, where my wife, Ezgi Ulusoy Aranyosi, had taken care of all the technology (computers, internet, air-conditioning), furniture, and renovations of the house in order to create the perfect working environment. Without her contribution, material and spiritual, this book would probably not have been completed.

Let me also thank the two anonymous referees for their constructive comments and their enthusiasm regarding the manuscript. Especially nowadays, when there are so many ideas on the market, so much competition to publish, and consequently so much divergence of opinion in the field, I feel lucky that two of my peers agreed about the merit of this book.

Last but not least, I would also like to thank Peter Ohlin, my editor from Oxford University Press, New York, for being always very prompt and kind in answering my queries during the review and production processes, as well as to photographer Alex Robciuc, who gave me permission to use his work for the cover of the book, and to graphic designer Adam Pękalski, who illustrated the monograph.

Finally, a few words about the book, its main ideas and structure, are in order. My approach in this monograph could easily be classified as part of the currently burgeoning "embodied mind" school or trend in contemporary philosophy of mind and cognitive science. Where it differs from most other works in this field is, I would say, in that (a) it offers a somewhat more focused view of embodiment via offering a conceptual role to the PNS as such in analyzing mental phenomena rather than keeping the discourse at the level of notions like "body" or "action", (b) it interprets the idea of the embodied mind not as most other philosophers, namely, representationally, as the body in the mind, but literally, namely, the mind as truly distributed over the body (in this sense, viz. of distinguishing if from most other popular approaches, I would rather call my approach "enminded body" than "embodied mind"), and (c) it relies a lot more on first-personal, phenomenological reflection when evaluating various theories about how things stand with the mind, without ending up in purely a priori conceptual analysis, but taking a lot of inspiration from empirical science (almost exclusively from neuroscience). Although most arguments I offer, and even the problems I raise in the book are, to my knowledge, new, the general points enumerated above, (a) to (c) are not totally absent from the current literature. I would especially like to express my intellectual debt to Shaun Gallagher's work, whose methodology and general approach to various issues was a great inspiration, even if the particular issues and debates he has been involved with are not present in this work. Temporally more distant and very important influences on my work in this book are Maurice Merleau-Ponty and James J. Gibson.

The four parts of the book seemed natural to me as a way to try to account for and develop the idea of the enminded body. The first part deals with more general and a priori issues, like how to formulate the hypothesis of the book, how to think of the phenomenal mind in a neuroscientific, reductionist manner, and how the Peripheral Mind Hypothesis can offer elegant solutions to some philosophical problems that need a priori reasoning. The second part discusses the boundaries of the mind, namely it argues against two types of externalism, Putnamian semantic externalism and the Extended Mind hypothesis of Chalmers and Clark. The originality of this part consists, in my view, in that at the end of the day both views get refined and clarified as a result of my discussion, even though I ultimately reject them. The third part is what I take as the most important and "meaty," namely an analysis of tactile and proprioceptive phenomena, heavily supported by empirical material and offering some novel arguments for taking peripheral nervous processes as constitutive of mental states rather than merely causal contributors to their existence. Finally, in the last part I discuss some general issues related to the emerging field of neuroethics, as well as two particular problems which seem to me to require reflection about the PNS, the problem of moral acceptability of abortion and the problem of moral acceptability of fulfilling physiologically healthy patient's requests for amputation or other functionally disruptive medical interventions.

István Aranyosi
October 12, 2012, Ankara

Abbreviations

ACh	Acetylcholine
BDD	Body Dismorphic Disorder
BIID	Body Integrity Identity Disorder
CNS	Central Nervous System
EC	Embodied Cognition
EEC	Embodied and Embedded Cognition
EED	extrinsic exteroceptive distance
EEE	extrinsic exteroceptive exterior
EEI	extrinsic exteroceptive interior
EEO	extrinsic exteroceptive orientation
GCT	Gate Control Theory of Pain
GID	Gender Identity Disorder
IPPD	intrinsic proprioceptive phenomenal distance
IPPE	intrinsic proprioceptive phenomenal exterior
IPPI	intrinsic proprioceptive phenomenal interior
IPPO	intrinsic proprioceptive phenomenal orientation
NMJ	neuromuscular junction
PMH	Peripheral Mind Hypothesis
PNS	Peripheral Nervous System
PP	"peripheral precedence"
PT	Pattern Theory
SFE	Stimulus Field Equivalence
ST	Specificity Theory
TES	transcranial electrical stimulation
TMS	transcranial magnetic stimulation
TR	transitional region

1

Margins of Me:
A Personal Story

A line from the hit song of 1970, "Big Yellow Taxi," by Joni Mitchell, reads: "Don't it always seem to go, that you don't know what you've got 'till it's gone." This means, of course, that you come to appreciate something you currently have only once you have lost it. This claim presupposes that, whatever you had, you were aware that you had it, but failed to value it. Yet some losses entail an even greater recognition: when you first notice upon losing something, *that you had something as such*. In such cases it is not merely a question of realizing a thing's value; even the fact of having it in your possession eludes you until you have it no longer. In other words, it is your failure to notice the thing while you have it that first enables you to "appreciate" it at its true value—once it is gone.

My example of such a case is that of a healthy peripheral nervous system (PNS). The PNS is the part of the nervous system of vertebrates that lies outside the brain and the spinal cord, and has the function of transmitting nerve impulses from the receptors located all over and inside the body to the central nervous system (CNS) consisting of the spinal cord and the brain, and from the CNS to the effectors, namely the skeletal and visceral muscles to be found in the body. The PNS is the primary interface between us and our environment. In a healthy PNS, its sensory part makes sure that we are sensitive to a wide range of stimuli via the receptor nerve cells found in the skin, the muscles, the mucosa of the nose, the retina of the eye,[1] and so on. Its motor part makes sure that we respond in the

---

[1] The retina, as well as the optic nerve, are officially classified in contemporary neuroscience as part of the CNS, based on their developmental origin as anatomical

right way to these stimuli, for instance, that we avoid noxious, pain-causing stimuli.

First, let me distinguish the case of the PNS from another type of case, namely, when in order for a good that you possess to perform optimally (i.e., as designed and at its peak), you are supposed not to pay attention to it, not to notice its working while it performs, lest you negatively interfere with its otherwise optimal performance. Most dynamic activities involving our bodies fit this description. When you play tennis, football, basketball, and so on, it is not at all advisable that you at any time start paying attention, say, visually, to how your feet or arms are moving, on pain of simply failing to optimally perform, if at all, the tasks involved in these activities. It is also plainly counterintuitive for us to start focusing on ourselves rather than on where the ball is, what speed it has, where the other players are located, how fast they move, and in which direction: the whole activity is not about contemplating what we ourselves are doing. These cases of involvement with the world, or phenomeno-logical immersion into the action have been noted before, for instance by Martin Heidegger,[2] or a psychologist like Mihály Csík-szentmihályi,[3] and it is part and parcel of the emerging, phenomeno-logical movement in the foundations of cognitive science, whose claims are understood within the tradition whose main figures are Edmund Husserl, Heidegger, and Maurice Merleau-Ponty.

However, while immersion or direct engagement with the world has as its conceptual counterpart the idea of a loss of oneself, or at least a weakened sense of oneself qua a self in relation to a world that is still external, the case of how the PNS connects the agent to the world is different in that it involves not *losing* oneself to the

---

units. However, from a neuro-functional point of view, it is more natural to consider them as part of the PNS. Hence, I use them as examples of PNS activity throughout, as from this work's perspective the neuro-functional criterion is more relevant than the anatomico-developmental.

[2]Heidegger, in several places throughout his *Being and Time*, talks about this involvedness via the idea of certain things being *ready-at-hand*, that is, possessing properties that depend on the activities in which these objects are properly used. It is essential to what these things are that they are used rather than contemplated.

[3]Hungarian psychologist Csíkszentmihályi (1990) proposed the notion of *flow* to explain what is going on during creative activities of people with high performance levels, like artists, musicians, academics, writers, although the notion has applicabil-ity for human activities as such. Flow is a state of complete focus, or complete absorp-tion with the activity at hand and the situation. Psychological components of flow include a loss of one's self-consciousness during the performance, a distorted subjec-tive sense of time, clear goals, focus, lack of awareness of bodily needs, and a balance between the level of the challenge presented by the activity and the level of the abil-ity of the performer.

world, but rather having an *intimate grip* on the world. In what follows I will appeal to my own experience of serious loss of some PNS function, and, of course, as any first-person account, it won't always be very precise, but I hope I can convey some points that are relevant to the guiding idea of this book.

On February 15, 2005, just four days after my public Ph.D. thesis defense, I was radiologically diagnosed with a very large neoplasm, a tumor occupying the middle of my chest, which later, after biopsy, turned out to be a case of Hodgkin's Lymphoma. Not long after, I started the treatment, which consisted of chemotherapy for about four months, followed by radiotherapy for three weeks. As part of the chemotherapy, based on the standard ABVD regimen, I was supposed to be administered Vinblastine, a *vinca* alkaloid obtained from the *Madagascar periwinkle*, which is a mitotic inhibitor (stops cell division). As it happened, because of a lack of Vinblastine at the oncology institute where I started my chemo, I was administered a chemical analogue, Vincristine. Both these *vinca* alkaloids are neurotoxic, but Vincristine is more frequently so and has more serious toxic effects on the PNS. The toxicity is dose-dependent, so if signs of serious nerve damage appear, administration of the drug is immediately discontinued. In milder cases it only interferes with motor functions related to refined motion, like undoing a shirt's button. In more severe cases it leads to peripheral neuropathy (paresthesias, loss of deep tendon reflexes), involving severe disturbance of the motor function. It can also become life-threatening when it affects the autonomic part of the PNS, leading sometimes to coma and respiratory arrest. It is also known that there are people with some pre-existing but latent nervous condition, who are more sensitive to Vincristine, and in whose case the drug should not be administered whatsoever, given its disruptive effects. Hence, the medical community nowadays recommends genetic testing of patients who are about to receive Vincristine, in order to avoid massive nerve damage (Perry and McKinney 2008: 631).

In my case it turned out that administering Vincristine was not a good idea. A few days after the second dose, and about eighteen days after the first one, I was leaving my apartment to take a walk downtown. I was walking downstairs, had already descended two floors, and when I had two or three more steps on the entrance stairs to reach the ground level I tumbled down. It was so quick and out of the blue that I couldn't explain why and how it happened. I looked for some object on the stairs that I could have tripped over, but there was nothing. A bit embarrassed, stood up and started walking. There was nothing to indicate that the problem was intrinsic to me. After a few minutes of a pleasant walk, I sat down at a computer in an Internet café to check my email, as my home connection wasn't working. I spent about half an hour sitting, browsing; I closed the browser, and I was about to get up and leave the place. I realized that I was not able to stand on my feet. I could raise my body a few centimeters, by pushing with my feet against the floor, but an extreme weakness invariably made me settle back on the seat. I immediately realized it had to do with Vincristine. During the month before my treatment started I had read a lot of medical literature related to my condition, including articles on the neurotoxic effects of *vinca* alkaloids, so I knew what to expect, and that sometimes serious motor effects can ensue. What I didn't expect was that the onset could be so sudden. Somehow I always assumed that if these neurological effects appeared, they would appear *gradually*, so one would be prepared in case more serious disturbance should follow. As the mild effects are numbness of the fingers and toes, as well as difficulties in executing precise, fine-grained motions, I assumed that that was how it was going to start, if I were to have such neurotoxicity at all. Yet, that wasn't the case.

After a few failed attempts to stand up quickly, I realized I had to do it slowly and by relying more on my arms. Finally, I could stand and walk slowly back home, which was about 200 meters from the café. The situation got worse and worse for the next six weeks, was stationary for a few weeks, and then began to improve. Meanwhile, of course, the administration of Vincristine was completely discontinued. In the first six weeks the denervation proceeded gradually from the toes to the ankles and middle of the legs, and also from the tip of my fingers to the middle of my forearms. So I ended up with a symmetrical, so-called glove-stocking type distribution of motor nerve damage. Sensory nerve fibers were unaffected. It took about two years to almost fully recover. Fortunately, the tumor also disappeared after about seven months, so I got cured of the main illness.

During this long time between the onset of the neuropathy and the almost full recovery, beyond the obvious malaise one is bound to go through, I had a chance to think about philosophical approaches to consciousness, sensory experience, and the self. The Ph.D. thesis I had completed and defended right before my tumor was identified was about the metaphysical mind-body problem, the issue of how a physicalist—someone who believes that everything that exists is physical and that all properties are either physical, or entailed by the totality of physical properties—is supposed to deal with phenomenal properties, with *what it is like to have* sensory experience. Actually, the presence of my tumor was established as a result of a standard X-ray screening I had to undergo in order to obtain an Australian long-term visa, before joining the Centre for Consciousness at the Australian National University, headed by David Chalmers, where I planned to continue working on consciousness as a postdoctoral fellow.

I knew of philosophers of mind who think that first-person data, phenomenological reflection based on how one subjectively feels or judges certain facts, are as important as third-person, objective data, when it comes to addressing philosophical problems about consciousness. I also knew of philosophers who started thinking about some philosophical problems based on some first-person experience. One example was my teacher, Howard Robinson, who once mentioned in class that he was prompted to write a book about perception by some puzzles that he thought were interesting, which arose in the context of his everyday experiences: for instance, the blurry image he used to get when putting on or removing eyeglasses, or the distortion of the visual field when he was gently pushing his eyeball from a side, or when one has an afterimage following an intense light stimulation of the eye. I used to think there was something unserious, even frivolous about such motivations to do philosophy, and, in general, that the idea of basing one's philosophy on subjective data is humbug, or at least dubious; and yet, and yet—I was now drawn to think about philosophical issues based on my condition.

One thing I realized during the period of severe peripheral neuropathy was the *déformation professionnelle* that we, philosophers of mind, have acquired by focusing so much on the brain and on the cranium when thinking about the self. It is in my opinion an extension of the Cartesian over-intellectualization of the mind. We could call it "cranialization." For instance, the literature on perception, when it comes to paradigmatic examples of perceptual phenomena, almost always focuses or starts from the visual case. Vision is somehow assumed to give the best picture of perceptual representation. And vision is of course something that involves the receptors in the eyes, which are in the cranium. There is an implicit bias here in favor of the perceiving self as paradigmatically residing, somehow, in the skull. The Cartesian tradition focuses on higher-order mental phenomena, like self-consciousness and abstract thinking. Through my experience I became aware of how much there is to the self inhabiting the extremities of the body, the limbs. My paradigmatic phenomenal self-perception was dependent on the sense of touch, on changes in gait, on kinesthesia, on the presence of the self at the extremities. The theoretical periphery has become a phenomenological center. It is important to stress that it was not merely that the body is present to the mind as a *body-image*—so the mind essentially perceives its attached body, but still the mind is thought of as confined to the brain—as some contemporary neuroscientists seem to think when in their more philosophical moments; here is, for instance Antonio Damasio (2010: 120):

> Messages from the skeletal muscles use different and fast-conducting kinds of nerve fibers—Aα and Aγ fibers—as well as different stations of the central nervous system all the way into the higher levels of the brain. The upshot of all this signaling is a multidimensional *picture of the body* in the brain *and, thus, in the mind.* (emphasis added)

As it happens, Damasio's latest (as I'm writing) book is replete with references to the brain as the seat of the mind, and, though bodily phenomena are taken seriously, they are supposed to fill in the role of *content* for what the brain/mind represents; here is another quote (Damasio 2010: 110):

> Because, as we have seen, brain maps are the substrate of mental images, map-making brains have the power of literally introducing the body as *content* into the mind process. Thanks to the brain, the body becomes a natural topic of the mind. (emphasis in original)

What I am talking about is very different. It is not the body as present to the mind in the representational sense, but the mind as such extending all over the body, and more exactly to all areas of the body that get innervated. This idea is better captured by a quote from Edward Rowland Sill, a lesser-known nineteenth-century American poet and essayist:

> The spinal cord runs along the back, with all its ganglia; the weight of the brain is well behind; yet *we* are not there. In other words, the curious thing is that we feel ourselves to be, not in the region where impressions are received and answered in the brain and spinal cord, but where they first meet the nerve-extremities. We seem to inhabit not the citadel, but the outer walls. At the point of peripheral expansion of the nerves of sense, where the outer forces begin to be apprehended by us as inner,—"in front," where the fingers feel, and the nose smells, and the eyes see—there, if anywhere, we feel ourselves to be. ([1900] 2001: 255) (emphasis in original)

And in the same vein, Maurice Merleau-Ponty observes that "the consciousness of the body invades the body, the soul spreads over all its parts, and behavior overspills its central sector" ([1945] 2002: 87).

These quotes present a quite different picture of the mind from either the Cartesian (or "textbook" Cartesian) soul in the body as a pilot in the cabin, or the contemporary neuroscientific picture of the mind as a brain possessing a body-image. The picture is rather of the mind as distributed in, or *infusing*, the body, thanks to the PNS. One could think of this metaphorically when talking about "my mind in my stomach when I am hungry," or "my mind in my finger when I feel pain," meaning only my minding my hunger and my pain, respectively, but I mean it literally: there is no reason to think that the stomach-mind (the part of the mind that is phenomenally located there) or the finger-mind is less of a mind than the brain-mind. In fact, the brain appears phenomenally mindless, doesn't it? Our modern and typically Western *everyday* way of thinking in terms of the brain as the seat of the mind is, in my view, clearly socially constructed in the sense of Berger and Luckmann (1966).

The first revelation I had about this was when, after receiving my chemotherapeutic infusion, I was sitting in the front seat and was preparing to get out of the car. I was supposed to lift my legs, one after the other, in order to step out. As my muscle weakness was serious, I had to grab the edge of my trousers with my hand, and help my leg muscles do the job; my hands were still working fine at that time. My impression was that the lower parts of my legs had become alien to me. It was the same impression as when you have a heavy object attached to your ankle which makes your muscles' flexion more difficult, except that now the heavy outer object was my own foot. And to that extent it ceased to proprioceptively feel like my own foot. My foot, or what used to be felt as my own foot before, has now become part of the *external world*; a piece of denervated, hence, alien flesh to be dragged around. Of course, visually the foot was mine; I could obviously see it and think of it as attached to the rest of my body, but when it comes to feeling your foot as yours, the visual ownership is fake ownership. The fact that visually and objectively the part-whole relation holding between your feet and yourself, its mereology, is not (too [much]) disrupted does not preclude whatsoever the clear disruption of its phenomenological mereology.

Incidentally, just a few months before, I had read a piece in a newspaper or magazine, in which the author was analyzing the phenomenon of online communities, in terms of whether such 'cyber-tribes' encourage social cohesion, or rather contribute to isolation and polarization within the larger social context. One of his examples of a weird and pernicious online community, which could not exist if internet had not been invented, was an online group whose membership is based on a shared psychiatric disorder, *apotemnophilia*. Those suffering from this disorder have a desire to have one or more of their limbs amputated, based on their sexual fantasies. In some of the more serious such cases, when the desire is very strong, the subjects suffer from a condition known as *Body Integrity Identity Disorder* (BIID), which makes them feel the relevant, otherwise completely healthy limb to be entirely alien to them, and seek the help of surgeons to perform an amputation. There are shocking case studies of this rare and fascinating disease, which indicate that some subjects show up at emergency rooms after self-inflicted injuries to the limb, in order to obtain emergency medical amputation. It is worth quoting from such a case study:

> One week later, the patient presented to the emergency department with bilateral lower-extremity pain, weakness, and swelling, along with 39.6°C fever and tachycardia. A repeat physical examination demonstrated 0/5 strength with dorsiflexion and plantar flexion of the feet bilaterally, along with bilateral, symmetrical erythema and edema of the lower extremities. Minor excoriations were noted on the patient's ankles, but no noticeable lacerations, ecchymoses, or puncture wounds were found. The patient was diagnosed with bilateral lower-extremity cellulitis as a complication of GBS (Guillain-Barré syndrome), and he was admitted to the neurology service for administration of intravenous antibiotics....
>
> At the surgeon's request to take the patient to the operating room, the patient requested bilateral below-the-knee amputations (BKAs) of his lower extremities. An orthopedic surgeon was consulted, and it was determined that amputation was not indicated, so the patient agreed to undergo bilateral incision and drainage of his lower extremities.
>
> Additional history was obtained from the patient's spouse, and she revealed that the patient's distal phalanges of the feet were missing because he had performed self-amputation with a tourniquet in 1999. The patient's spouse further confessed that the patient had had a past fascination with amputations, and she had previously discovered him placing tourniquets around his lower extremities at various times. It was concluded that his bilateral neuropathy and cellulitis of the lower extremities were due to self-induced ischemia with tourniquets. The patient was diagnosed with apotemnophilia and transferred to the psychiatric service for further evaluation and treatment. (Bensler and Paauw 2003: 674 75)

I will talk more about apotemnophilia and BIID in the last chapter of this book, devoted to some topics in neuroethics, and about the notion of embodiment in general in chapters 6, 7, and 8. The reason I mentioned such cases now is to point out that when first reading about them I found it hard to empathize with these patients, but now I had a different perspective, which, except for the pathological components, made me realize to some extent what it must be like to feel your limbs to be foreign.

In my case, of course, the prevailing sentiment was that of the loss of something whose absence made me now realize how important it is when present—just like in the Joni Mitchell song this introductory essay started with. That the opposite must be true of a BIID sufferer is nicely brought out by an episode of the BBC TV series *Casualty* in which a woman loses her leg; it gets destroyed by a train. Her behavior and attitude are bizarre, as she were unfazed by what has happened—just *unlike* in the Joni Mitchell song. She is later diagnosed with BIID.

I had a similar experience with my hands. The onset of the neuropathy at that level occurred a few weeks after the one at the level of the feet. Within a few days my fingers got bent, my hand assumed an inward bending, with the palms turned toward the forearm, and an extreme muscle weakness ensued, which made me unable to grasp even a spoon. Again, my hands felt like a foreign object attached to my "real hand," that is to whatever was left in terms of innervation that could still serve more or less as an ersatz hand when it comes to hand-specific motion. I was soon to adapt to the situation by involuntarily learning how to execute hand-involving motor tasks based partly on visual information and partly on the proprioception of the whole arm. For instance, pushing the start button of the TV set, or of the computer, or turning the light on/off by pushing a button, were actions that I would soon learn to execute with more or less precision. The recipe was first to visually fixate on where the button is, and then to throw the whole hand, with its bent and weary fingers, toward it through the air, by using the large muscles of the arm, in such a way that one of the fingers would land exactly on the button and push it. The push itself, once the finger has successfully landed, was based on the action of the large muscles of the arm and the pure mechanics of solidity and the limits that the joints have in bending, and almost complete lack of any muscle contribution from the hand.

I learnt similar tricks for the feet, although that was painful. In the early days I wasn't yet used to the new conduction patterns and speeds in the motor fibers of my legs, so I fell over a few times in the house, injuring myself, because I 'misunderstood' the time I need for my legs to react to the decision of moving them. One such case was when someone rang the doorbell and I immediately wanted to proceed to the door, but my legs were slower than how my will expected them to react, so I fell and injured my knee and my ankle. During those times I underwent several sessions of (quite long and tiring, and somewhat painful) nerve conduction tests and EMG (electromyography) set up by my neurologist, who was writing a Ph.D. thesis on chemo-toxicity induced peripheral neuropathies. I learnt that my damage was axonal, that is, it was only the axons that got severed by the chemical attack, which otherwise left the cell bodies of the neurons intact; this gave me hope for the future recovery of the fibers. The nerve conduction tests showed a reduction of the nerve conduction speed in all the main motor nerve fibers in the legs; some were conducting at half speed, others even slower. There is a direct positive correlation between the extent of the damage (i.e., thickness of a fiber after injury) and its conduction speed. The test for sensory fibers showed that those were not affected. Heat, soft touch, and pain stimuli elicited the normal patterns of neural activity.

The reason I said earlier that the mind is neither the Cartesian, highly intellectualized, cranium-confined firm-and-frozen ego, nor the self-effaced, world-immersed, flowing, field-like non-thingy occurrence, is that even though I was feeling my limbs to be alien to myself, that did not mean that I felt them to be *disconnected*. Rather, they were intimately connected, yet, merely *connected* to me, and not phenomenologically proper parts of myself. The mind-world boundary seems to have moved from the skin/environment junction to the innervated/denervated junction within the body. So part of the body has become external to the mind, or 'de-minded'. It was only then that I started thinking about the mind as really present throughout the body rather than as merely containing a body-image or being informed by the body. The most obvious case that used to bring about this feeling was related to gait. Naturally, the nerve damage has distorted my gait; walking was very risky and insecure. More importantly, the new perspective on walking made me think of the mind-world connection in the normal case as of an intimate grip on the external environment, on whatever felt or presented itself as external to myself. That kind of intimate grip was now experienced between myself and my lower legs; they were connected tightly, so that they could be manipulated, moved in a rough manner, but they at the same time felt external to the mind or self. For instance, walking with damaged peripheral nerves provided the impression of no important differences between stepping on hard concrete and stepping on a soft carpet. Stepping on almost any kind of surface felt pretty much the same: pushing against a soft and unsteady surface, with a lot of muscles all over the legs tiring themselves in a concerted and seemingly chaotic effort to compensate for balance. I was toddling on a ubiquitous ocean of cotton rags embroiled with a motley assortment of scattered and jagged terrain, jeering back at the struggling neural flotsam that was left in the legs to keep the whole body edifice in good balance.

This intimate grip on the world can be extended to other sense modalities. There is a peripheral presence of the mind in every part of the body that gets innervated, and these peripheral parts of the mind are no less central than the processing center, which is the brain. The fact that the brain is the processing center does not entail in any way that it must be a phenomenological center. On the contrary, I think that we have every reason to think of the peripheral mind as phenomenologically and objectively part and parcel of what we used to think of as the mind or the self. Doing so, as it will become apparent in the following chapters, will provide many new and elegant solutions to philosophical puzzles related to the notions of mind and body. The ears, the eyes, the soft visceral tissues, the skin, and so on are all minded. I noted earlier that the mind, according to the picture I try to advance here, is multiply located. What I mean by 'multiply located' is not the same as 'scattered'. It is not that the mind has parts that are co-located in the ordinary sense with parts of the body. What I mean is closer to the sui generis notion of recurrence that we find in the writings of metaphysicians who are committed to realism about universals. Universals, like redness, tallness, sweetness, and so on, are said to be multiply located or recurrent entities, in the sense that they are entirely present in all their instances regardless of the time and place these instances are to be found. So, for instance, the same redness is present at the same time in two spatially separated red objects. This notion of recurrence is puzzling in some ways because it does not allow universals to be located in the same ordinary physical way as particulars (objects and events) are. The relation of *being co-located with*, in the ordinary physical sense, is transitive—if *a* is co-located with both *b* and *c*, then *b* and *c* are themselves co-located—but the sense in which a universal is co-located with something does not satisfy transitivity: redness is co-located with a red apple and with a red bag, yet the apple and the bag are not co-located. The universal, by its nature, is co-located with objects that are not themselves co-located; it is entirely present in diverse places.

Now, of course, many philosophers are skeptical about the notion of a universal precisely because of such a weird way for universals to be located, which, these philosophers argue, should not even be called 'location'. But a weakness in one domain becomes a strength in another. It is well known how hard it is to think of our consciousness as located somewhere. For one, it is not thingy enough to be located in the same way as ordinary things, particulars, are; and yet, it is undeniable that while being conscious we experience consciousness as being present. Where? Well, no one, including philosophers or neuroscientists who insist that the self is the brain, really has a knock-down argument for one location or another. Yet others think that consciousness is rather characterized by non-locality, on a par with the notion of non-locality in quantum physics (e.g., Clarke 1995). A great psychologist, unfortunately largely forgotten in academia at least, Julian Jaynes, wrote that although we tend to immediately locate our mind or self when prompted to do so, and we usually point to our heads, somewhere behind the eyes, there is strictly speaking no reason whatsoever to do so:

> [W]e are continually inventing these spaces in our own and other people's heads, knowing perfectly well that they don't exist anatomically; and the location of these 'spaces' is indeed quite arbitrary. The Aristotelian writings, for example, located consciousness or the abode of thought in and just above the heart, believing the brain to be a mere cooling organ since it was insensitive to touch or injury. And some readers will not have found this discussion valid since they locate their thinking selves somewhere in the upper chest. For most of us, however, the habit of locating consciousness in the head is so ingrained that it is difficult to think otherwise. But, actually, you could, as you remain where you are, just as well locate your consciousness around the corner in the next room against the wall near the floor, and do your thinking there as well as in your head. Not really just as well. For there are very good reasons why it is better to imagine your mind-space inside of you, reasons to do with volition and internal sensations, with the relationship of your body and your 'I'. (Jaynes [1976] 2000: 45 46)

Here is the same point made a hundred years earlier by Sill:

> [T]here is one point concerning our felt location which I think we are all sure of. It is the one brought out so deliciously by the dear little girl in "Punch." "You ought to tie your own apron-strings, Mabel!" says one of those irresistible young women of Du Maurier's. "How can I, Aunty?" is the reply. "I'm in front, you know!" ([1900] 2001: 255)

Maybe, when it comes to consciousness, we should not think of location in the ordinary sense in which particulars are located, but in the sense in which universals are supposed to be 'located'. The idea can be brought out in the context of another, independent discussion in philosophy, namely, the problem of how to understand the unity of consciousness. What is it that makes distinct experiences at some time the experiences of the same conscious subject? What explains co-consciousness? Instances of co-consciousness are all over the place. Imagine yourself walking on a road, while talking on your cell phone, watching the scenery before your eyes, hearing the distant sound of a train's horn, smelling the fresh bread that is being baked as you pass by the bakery, and being hungry—all at the same time. What makes all these quasi-simultaneously occurring experiences co-conscious, that is, the experiences of one unitary mind?

It is tempting for philosophers with a naturalistic inclination to start thinking about a physical place where all these experiences 'come together', so they appear as co-conscious, and that will be, according to these philosophers, the brain. My picture is quite different. Experiences do not *come* together; they *are* together all the way. The picture is not that of a bunch of rivers that end up flowing into the same sea or ocean, so that it is the fact of flowing into *the same sea or ocean* that makes them unitary in some way. The picture is that of a sea or ocean, very much unlike our real seas and oceans, flowing out into a myriad of branches and a myriad of other branches flowing back into it, such that *the whole system* composed of the ocean and the in and out flowing streams count as one system. The way a system is present in more than one location is not merely by having its parts in different places; a system *qua system* is present across various locations in space or time by its parts at those locations interacting with all the other parts in the way the system requires in order to really count as a system. This is the picture I have in mind when thinking about the nervous system composed of the CNS and the PNS. It is not that the PNS is merely a transmitter of neural 'messages' that come together in the brain to form a unitary consciousness at the phenomenal level, but rather the PNS is the structure that ensures that the body is *minded*, the structure that makes it possible for consciousness to be multiply located all over and inside the body. For experiences to be co-conscious is for them to be processes integrated with each other within the patterns of the same nervous system, CNS and PNS. If there are hard cases, for instance, thought experiments involving someone's brain being connected to someone else's limbs, these cases boil down to the question of how to individuate nervous systems themselves. If my brain gets connected to the PNS of another person, while that other person's PNS gets disconnected from her brain, then in fact that PNS is not hers anymore; it becomes mine, and so it is my mind that suffuses her body, even though in many other ways (blood circulation, metabolism, etc.) those limbs are still hers. Phenomenologically, or as far as mindedness is concerned, those limbs are mine, because now I am the one who can use them as a way to have an intimate grip on the world.

To return to the idea of understanding the location of consciousness on the model of the recurrence of universals, my main hypothesis will be that sensory states are present both at the level of the CNS and that of the PNS, and more exactly that it is constituted by CNS and PNS processes. Now, the presence of consciousness in the body could be understood on the model of universals *simpliciter*, but I think a better picture is given by the notion of a distributional universal or property, a notion proposed by Josh Parsons (2004). A distributional property is, intuitively, a way of filling in or "painting" an extended object with some quality or qualities. To understand what we are talking about we should give a few examples: *being polka-dotted* (which is a color pattern distribution on a surface), *being hot at one end and cold on the other* (which is a way for heat to be distributed over an object), *having a rough texture* (which is a way crystals are distributed within a material), *having a uniform density throughout* (which is a way to distribute density throughout a solid object or a fluid).

Distributional properties are the best picture of the way I like to think of sensory states in this book, for two reasons. One is phenomenological, that is, related to how consciousness feels like or appears from the first-person perspective, and I have already touched upon it. Consciousness feels distributed throughout the body, and this is immediately apparent when we consider co-conscious states, like the ones described above. Although these co-conscious states are different in kind, as they are based on distinct sense modalities, they still appear phenomenally states of the same consciousness. The second reason for thinking of conscious states as involving distributional properties is neurophysiological. As will be made clear later in the book, sensory states, like pain, are not accounted for by a definite place in the brain, but as a continuous interaction among the peripheral nerve fibers, the spinal cord, and several areas in the brain. This means that a neuroscientific account of these states will involve large areas of both the CNS and the PNS, and the state itself is therefore most naturally understood as a distributional property of the nervous system, where what is distributed is electrical activity.

Of course, the issues I have so far mentioned indiscriminately— phenomenal self-presence or being-there, location of consciousness, co-consciousness, system presence—are really distinct problems and have been discussed independently, but in the context of the corticocentrist prejudice I have pointed out above, which will later be exemplified in various chapters, they are different ways to make my main point to the effect that there is a good case to challenge this prejudice.

Back to my story. In short, within several months of the onset of the neuropathy a slow process of improvement started, first at the level of the hands, then, a few weeks later, at the level of the legs. I was testing myself every day for what I was or was not able to execute, so first I realized that my hand's grip had improved; I was able to hold a spoon, for instance, and later, when my legs started improving, I was able to hold onto the balustrade when trying to walk downstairs. As far as the legs are concerned, every day brought a small success: standing up by myself, walking to the window by myself, jumping up a couple of centimeters and landing safely, without my legs collapsing at the level of the knees, and finally being able to walk downstairs by holding onto the balustrade. This last achievement was quite important for me, as I remember its exact date, September 15, 2005, when I walked sixteen steps downstairs and up again.

Then things got much better, even professionally. In April 2006, with more than a year's delay, I finally made it to Australia, where I spent a whole year at the ANU's Philosophy Program at the Research School of Social Sciences—probably the greatest place on Earth for a philosopher to be. My neuropathy wasn't completely gone yet, but in August 2006 I was already able to run a few tens of meters on the shores of Kioloa Beach, 150 kilometers West of Canberra, on the South Pacific Ocean, where ANU has a campus, and where I had a chance to participate in the indubitably greatest two philosophy conferences in my life thus far. Let me use this space for thanking David Chalmers for making my great Australian experience, and many other things in my professional career, possible.

This book on the peripheral mind has been at the back of my mind for years, but it was only in 2011 that I thought I felt ready to actually approach this topic in writing. I hope it will at least offer some new insights into some old philosophical problems surrounding the life of the mind, which could be developed in the future, so the reader will, hopefully, not be disappointed.

Part I

Minds and Nerves

2

A Philosophical Hypothesis

In this chapter my aim is to make clear what the *Peripheral Mind Hypothesis* (PMH), the main hypothesis of the book, is and to present some empirical data on the Peripheral Nervous System (PNS). I will explain what it means that PMH is a philosophical hypothesis and how it is related to theory building in cognitive neuroscience, as exemplified by visual awareness research. Finally, I will also consider the issue of how to adjudicate between approaches that view conscious experience as an end product somewhere in the brain and my own approach, which takes PNS and CNS components responsible for experience as constituents of it. Whereas this chapter focuses more on neuroscience, the rest of the book will deal with philosophical applications of PMH.

I. PMH as a Philosophical Hypothesis

You might think that there is no place for philosophy when it comes to an empirical domain like cognitive neuroscience. Ever so much nowadays there are, indeed, philosophers who, paradoxically enough, are pushing such a claim. They start from the reasonable idea that philosophy should be consistent and inspired by empirical research, rather than based purely on armchair reflection, and end up with the unreasonable view that philosophy should be purged of armchair, conceptual reflection completely. Of course, given that this purging is not in fact possible, and not only in philosophy, but also in scientific theorizing itself, some of these philosophers end up with a purely rhetorical embracement of "science" and rejection of "traditional philosophy." As Timothy Williamson has recently pointed out, there are many philosophers *claiming* that philosophy should be "scientific" or "naturalistic," but not all of those actually move beyond the rhetoric and *do* some empirically founded philosophy:

> Many contemporary philosophers have some sympathy for crude empiricism, particularly when it goes under the more acceptable name of "naturalism." However, that sympathy sometimes has little effect on their philosophical practice: they still philosophize in the grand old manner, merely adding naturalism to their list of *a priori* commitments. (2007: 1–2)

There is plenty of space for traditional philosophy in cognitive neuroscience, especially in theory building. I will exemplify this claim by reference to recent research on visual awareness, which involves a lot of purely conceptual issues, including philosophical methodology and intuition-based argumentation by neuroscientists themselves. Before that, however, let me formulate the main claim of this book.

The main claim of this book is that we could think of the mind as constitutively incorporating not only the brain processes but also the ones that take place at the level of the PNS. I will develop this claim a bit, but first let me explain the idea that we *could* think of the mind this way. When I say that we could think of the mind this way, I mean two things. One is that it is not conceptually incoherent to think of it this way. The other is that the hypothesis does not conflict with theories in cognitive neuroscience. There are further questions that arise. Is the hypothesis *supported* by empirical data in cognitive neuroscience? Do I have an argument for a stronger claim to the effect that we *must* think of the mind this way? It would be nice if there were definite positive answers to these questions. But there aren't. However, this is not because there is something wrong with the hypothesis, but because of its nature. The hypothesis is a philosophical one, whose virtues are not so much its purportedly being explanatory of existing data, or exclusively explanatory of other data, or predictive of future data. Its virtues are its benefits as far as arguments, intuitions, and elegant solutions to classic puzzles in the philosophy of mind are concerned. We will see these philosophical benefits from the next chapter on. What I want to stress at this point is that being a philosophical hypothesis, PMH is mainly useful for solving extant and future philosophical conundrums. It is on a par with other cases in philosophy, for instance, ontological hypotheses, like: the A- and B-theory of time, the psychological criterion for personal identity, the supervenience of everything on microphysical facts (physicalism), and so on. Such hypotheses are to be tested in terms of philosophical costs and benefits, even though they might have empirical basis and implications. Of course, I will appeal to several findings in empirical science that are clearly relevant to the issues I will discuss.

This being said let us return to the claim that PMH makes and clarify it. The way I have enunciated it, the claim is too rough. We need some qualifications regarding each component concept that figures in it. First, let us take the term "mind." The concept of a mind refers to the collection of mental states, events, and properties that a conscious being possesses over a period of time. I do not mean to apply PMH to the mind in its entirety, but only to cases of mental items that typically causally involve sensorimotor loops; hence, they causally involve the PNS. All the sensory systems, like vision, tactile experience, auditory experience, proprioception, gustatory and olfactory experience, mechanoception, equilibrioception, nociception (perception of pain), are like this, and they comprise a large portion of the conscious human mind. There are mental items that do not *typically* involve the PNS and also ones that involve it atypically. From the first category we can mention memory, reasoning, imagination, whereas from the second one we can mention dream experience. So what I focus on are sensory systems and their associated conscious experiences.

Next, the claim is that the peripheral components that are involved in sensory experiences are not merely causally involved in the generation of experience, but constitutively so. Everyone agrees that the PNS is a causal component in the nervous process that is correlated with sensory experience. But it is only recently that some philosophers of cognitive science have put forward the constitution thesis, though not exactly the way I put it in this book. A number of authors, like O'Regan and Noë (2001), Noë (2004), Myin and O'Regan (2009), and the classics Varela, Thompson, and Rosch (1991) and Lakoff and Johnson (1999), argue that some peripheral events are constitutive of human mentality, not merely causally effective in bringing about it. While all these authors stress the efferent pathways as essential to conscious experience, that is, they posit action as constitutive of perception, I stress the afferent component, namely, the sensory parts of the PNS as constitutive of rather than causing experience. As we will see later, in chapter 8, there are a number of important differences between all these views, gathered under the name *Embodied Cognition* (EC), and the views I propose here. There is one difference, however, that I would like to stress here. It is that whereas the theorists involved in the EC research agenda have been preoccupied with defending their theses against criticism from the "classicist" side, that is, from those who are skeptical that there is need for a second generation of cognitive science, radically different from the classic approaches, or from those who think that the EC approach is not that revolutionary after all, I am more preoccupied with mapping the philosophical benefits of my thesis. This has not properly been done, in my opinion; hence, the hoped-for novelty of the approach in this book.

So let me reformulate my main claim so as to reflect what has been said so far:

> (PMH) Conscious mental states typically involved in sensory processes are partly constituted by subprocesses occurring at the level of the PNS.

What the hypothesis says is that typical sensory conscious states have the PNS activity as their constitutive parts. One would be tempted to add to the end of PMH: "whenever these PNS processes are present," in order to avoid the stronger claim that being constitutive parts, *exactly the same* PNS processes are present in all logically possible worlds in which the mental state is present. Philosophers typically do not want to exclude that a mental state could be brought about via direct stimulation of the brain. I also think that direct stimulation of the brain can create sensory and perceptual states, but see the corollary below.

I have already excluded dreams from this hypothesis, as the connection between the sensory states in dreams and the PNS is much less tight in actual fact. There are, of course, triggering peripheral causes of specific sensory dream contents, but these are not correlated in the typical way. Yet, even in the case of dreams, when certain peripheral or central stimuli together with memory contents and access generate the dreamed sensory state, one could argue that evolutionary and developmental facts that were responsible for the regulation of typical waking state counterparts of these sensory states explain why dream contents are as they are,[1] in which case

---

[1] There are in effect theorists arguing that the role of dreaming is to train the sensorimotor system, hence, dreaming is indirectly connected to the adaptive and developmental needs of the waking state sensorimotor mechanisms. See Blumberg 2010.

PMH would apply even to dreams in an indirect way, by tracing the explanation back to such evolutionary and developmental histories.

The hypothesis is, at the same time, strong enough, as I add a further claim, which I take as a corollary to it; call it *Stimulus Field Equivalence* (SFE), or, to appeal to an informal way to put it, *The Eye for an Eye Principle*:

> (SFE/Eye for an Eye) Conscious mental states typically involved in sensory processes can conceivably successfully be brought about by direct stimulation of the brain, and in all such cases the utilized stimulus field will be in the relevant sense equivalent to the actual PNS or part of it thereof.

The relevant sense of equivalence in each case is given by what we know empirically about how the external stimuli are turned into neural signals by the appropriate transducers, like the peripheral nerve endings in the retina in the case of vision, or those in the olfactory epithelium in the nasal cavity. Relevant here are the field-like or topological properties of the transduction and the further afferent projection. For instance, we know very well that in the visual system there is a phenomenon of *retinotopy*, that is, a topographical mapping from the retina to the visual cortex. The early cortical visual areas, like the primary visual cortex, V1, were possible to chart using fMRI due to the fact that retinotopy involves a projection of the neighboring regions on the retina onto neighboring regions in V1. This mapping is preserved, although with distortions and lateral displacement, at the next cortical levels, V2, V3, V3A, and V4. Retinotopy preserves the spatial qualitative relations of the retina whenever the latter is stimulated in the appropriate way (Sereno et al. 2001; Arcaro et al. 2011). Similar topographical ideas apply to the organization of color stimuli within the nervous system. Although most studies have been done on the visual cortex, and the visual system is the best know as of today, homologous topographical properties of the PNS-CNS connection are supposed to be present in other systems too, for instance, in the auditory system (Chevillet et al. 2011), and even in systems that were traditionally thought as failing to involve maplike organization of their stimulus fields, like olfaction (Mombaerts et al. 1996).

This empirical knowledge is relevant to the philosophical point that my corollary, SFE, makes, namely, that the PNS is constitutive part of mental states in that any direct stimulation of the cortex directed at re-creating a current experience will have to also re-create the topographical mapping properties of the PNS-CNS connection. It is this sense in which any successful stimulation of the cortex will ultimately have to involve stimulus fields that will be equivalent to how the PNS actually structures environmental or internal information.[2]

The evidence for my claim is partly empirical, partly thought experimental, and hence a priori. If you try to imagine how exactly an experience could be created by direct stimulation of the cortex, say, via transcranial magnetic stimulation (TMS), you will at some point rely on the data that the actual PNS provides the cortex with, otherwise you cannot claim to have credibly described a case of such alleged re-creation of an experience. Philosophers all too easily neglect the details when it comes to thought experiments. The brain in a vat is supposed to be a brain whose experiences are exactly as mine, but they are artificially created by a computer via direct cortex stimulation. I will put my thought experiment to use in both chapters 4 and 7, and our corollary, SFE, will prove to address philosophical issues in a novel way. For now, let us keep in mind that SFE is not some abstract metaphysical principle, but it is actually supported by what we know about the nervous system and by intuitions based on this knowledge to the effect that direct brain stimulation should not be taken as bringing about the relevant experience in a deus ex machina fashion, as philosophers negligently assume it to happen, but it will be constrained by actual facts about the PNS-CNS connection. As a matter of actual empirical fact, we don't yet know much about how exactly, by what neural mechanisms direct stimulation creates experiences. Recent studies on transcranial electrical stimulation (TES) of the cortex suggest, much in line with my hypothesis, that even in a case one might have thought to be paradigmatically exclusively brain-involving, namely, generation of phosphenes (experiences of flashes of light without light entering the eye), the origin of these is retinal (Schutter and Hortensius 2010; Kar and Krekelberg 2012). Of course, as I mentioned in the introduction, the retina is considered as part of the brain, but that is more like a convention based on the fact that the retina originates in the primitive brain tissue formed in the early stages of embryonic

---

[2]The point is made, more generally, that precise re-creation of the experience of the external world will have to involve the peripheral reconstruction of a body, with all its relevant components, not only neural but hormonal and anatomical, among others, by Damasio (1994: ch. 10), Gallagher (2005: ch. 6), and Thompson (2007: 240–42).

development. However, functionally, which is the relevant criterion from the point of view of this book, the retina, as well as the optic nerve, are peripheral neural components.

Against this, philosophers will typically appeal to conceivability as "proof of possibility." Indeed, one objection raised against my "Eye for an Eye" principle, during the draft stage of this book, was that a phenomenal copy of an actual sensory state could come into being in a brain completely randomly; there is no logical necessity in having to voluntarily stimulate such a brain in order to make an experience actual, even though empirically my principle looks very credible. Consider that I am in pain right now. The allegedly conceivable scenario of my objector consists of two claims: (i) that whatever state my brain is actually in right now could be replicated by a brain, via a random event, and (ii) I would be in pain in that scenario. I agree with claim (i). I don't see why the same neural processes, electrical activity, neurotransmitter release and reuptake, and so on could not just pop into existence out of nothing, without any PNS-like structure. However, claim (ii) is nothing else but a denial of my main hypothesis, namely that PNS components are constitutive of mental states. My objector cannot claim that the alleged intuition about (ii) is completely pre-theoretical. On the contrary, it must assume that mental states are located exclusively in the brain; and this I deny. The objector could insist and say that there is no intuition that sensory phenomenal states are not exclusively located in the brain. But then I would challenge her and ask whether there is any intuition that such states are brain-bound; and if brain-bound, why not located at a specific area of the brain? And further, why not bound to an even smaller area, or even to one single neuron? Now the objector will probably reply that one neuron is not enough for realizing a phenomenal state, but more structure is needed. Then I ask: How much structure? And why should that necessary structure stop at the level of the brain stem? In truth, there is no such thing as an "intuitive boundary" of a sensory state. That most philosophers take such states as brain-bound is not an intuition, but a prejudice.

II   PMH and the Case of Visual Awareness Research

As I have stated before, philosophical speculation is not alien to neuroscience itself. The theoretical debates on visual awareness are such an example of scientific endeavor with heavily philosophical underpinnings, in which theorists are not shy to appeal to intuitions, just as philosophers do. The question of visual awareness, as it is explicitly presented in the neuroscience literature, is: Which part of the brain enters visual awareness directly? Or: where in the brain is visual awareness ultimately located? If I am right, these questions are loaded with a false presupposition, namely, that there is such a place in the brain. Another corollary of PMH that I would like to state here is a reductionist one, to the effect that experiential states are identical to total processes involving the PNS and the CNS. The processes of feedforward and feedback (more on these below) constitute or are identical to experiences. Hence, if I am right in my philosophical hypothesis, then the quest for a *cortical* area that "enters consciousness directly," or "of which we are directly aware," or "which constitutes our consciousness" is misguided.

To cut to the chase, here is a quote from two prominent theorists in cognitive neuroscience, Francis Crick and Christopher Koch, in which what they argue against is precisely my hypothesis, PMH, and their argument has a characteristically philosophical flavor, because they appeal to our ordinary intuitions:

> Some readers may find our suggestion counterintuitive, partly because for many years V1 was the only visual cortical area that was worked on extensively. We would ask them: do you believe that you are directly aware of the activity in your retina? (Of course, without your retinae, you cannot see anything) If you do not believe this, what is the argument that you are directly aware of the neural activity in V1? (1995: 122)

Let us first note the oddity of formulating the issue in terms of "direct awareness of one's neural activity" (more on this in chapter 7). Second, let us put this quote in the larger context of the theoretical debates about visual awareness and then analyze the argument. The story starts with a debate during the 1970s about whether visual processing at cortical level is serial or parallel. Serial processing means that the information transmitted via nerve impulses undergoes processing (selection, integration, etc.) in only one cortical area at once, whose output is then projected to another area, and so on; so what we get is the simplest hierarchical model of processing based on serial processing involving one area at a time. Yet, later, evidence accumulated showing that visual processing is not completely serial, but parallel at various levels of the hierarchy of areas. Parallel processing means that the information is projected to and processed by various disjoint areas at the same time. However, the theoretical focus moved to the very idea of a hierarchy of visual areas. Van Essen and Maunsell (1983) were the first to state the currently used criterion for constructing a hierarchy of visual areas that is orthogonal to the issue of whether at some point in the trajectory of the nerve impulse processing is serial or parallel. They defined three types of connections, which are today standardly used by neuroscience to distinguish higher from lower areas: feedforward connections, feedback connections, and lateral connections. They are distinguished based on the laminar distribution of their cells of origin and of their axonal terminations. Laminar distribution means the level of depth in the cortex from which these connections originate and the level of depth where they project. Forward or ascending connections were defined, on the model of thalamocortical pathways, as the ones that originate from superficial layers and terminate most densely in layer IV. Feedback or descending connections were defined as ones that originate from both superficial and deep layers and terminate most densely in outside layer IV. Finally, lateral connections were defined as the ones conforming to an intermediate pattern of approximately equal density of origins and terminations in all layers. Higher levels were assigned to areas according to whether the area is immediately following a feedforward connection, and areas that are connected by lateral connections were assigned the same level. This leads to six hierarchical levels for the twelve visual areas.

Around the same time, David Marr, in his celebrated *Vision* (1982), elaborated a theory of visual processing that fit very well with the hierarchical model of visual areas. Marr's theory was based on a serial filtering process executed at each stage of the visual hierarchy, so it was in the serialist paradigm. The anatomical hierarchy based on the three types of connection has become the basis for a functional model of the visual system. According to Marr, the visual information was supposed to pass through three stages: (i) the primal sketch, locally computed at lower levels V1 and V2 as a 2D sketch of the visual scene presented as a retinal image,[3] (ii) the $2D^{1/2}$ representation, and (iii) the final 3D representations, supposed to be computed at higher levels. The model is serial because the increase in complexity of the information follows the direction of feedforward connections. Also, Marr's theory is considered by some philosophers the paradigmatic Cartesian, or standard cognitive science

---

[3]What is meant by "retinal image" is a pattern of electromagnetic stimulation, which, according to Marr, is not yet a representation. It becomes a representation as a result of higher order filtering at various cortical levels.

(Rowlands 2010: 26), in that it presupposes that the conscious mind is located somewhere in the brain and that processing is based on manipulation and transformation of internal representations.

Finally, we reach the debate over visual awareness, where there are two main views that have taken shape. One is a serialist approach, based on Marr's legacy, according to which the final conscious percept is to be found at the top of the Van Essen-Maunsell hierarchy. The above quote from Crick and Koch is an example of such theory.[4] Let us go back to the quote and try to see what the argument against V1, the primary visual field, being the seat of the conscious percept is. Well, it is apparent that the argument is one that philosophers typically use: an argument from intuition and analogy. We could represent it more formally as follows:

1. It is ordinarily counterintuitive to think that the processes at the level of your retina directly enter the conscious visual percept you have.
2. If 1, then it is equally counterintuitive that processes at the level of the primary visual cortex V1 directly enter your conscious visual percept.
3. Hence, we should place the visual percept at the highest levels in the cortical hierarchy.

As it happens, I think this is a quite bad argument. There are good objections to both premises, and on top of that the conclusion does not follow, so the argument, as it stands, is invalid. I won't spend too much time on this, because I want to focus on the fact that the argument has presuppositions that make it irrelevant to my PMH hypothesis. So I will very briefly mention some objections to the premises and why the argument is invalid. The objection to premise 1 is that it is not an ordinary intuition that the percept is not at the level of the retina, even if ordinary, nonexpert people would have this intuition. It is an intuition based on an interpretation or misinterpretation of what neuroscience has discovered about the brain. I am sure that even as close to our time as four hundred years ago both ordinary people and scientists would have found it very intuitive that the conscious visual percept occurs at the level of the eye per se, not even at the level of the retina. I also think that the current ordinary seeming intuition that Crick and Koch are pushing is based on a vague idea and a misinterpretation of neuroscientific

[4] Another example is Rees et al. 2002.

findings. Where the percept is located is precisely the issue here, so Crick and Koch's alleged anti-retinal intuition is a subtle way of begging the question, as if we already know where neuroscience has placed the percept in the nervous system. The objection to the second premise is that the conditional it states is based on a dodgy analogy. The reason why ordinary people find it "crazy" to place the percept at the level of the retina is because they think it must be at the cortical level. Now that reason does not work to distinguish cortical areas V1 or V2 from another area, like V4. So the analogy breaks down when the intuition is tested cortico-cortically. Finally, the argument is invalid, because what follows from the two premises is only that the percept is located at a level higher than V4. Crick and Koch are not alone in arguing this way. Here is a quote from Alan Cowey, which is based on the same intuition about the retina as unfit for containing the percept:

> When any part of the primary visual cortex in man is destroyed, the patient has a visual field defect in which he is clinically blind. Although this does not necessarily prove that conscious visual percepts are created there—*after all, we are blind if the eyes are destroyed, but no one suggests that visual consciousness is created there*—it does indicate the importance of V1 to visual awareness, especially as destruction of no other visual area produces phenomenal blindness. (2005: 1199) (emphasis added)

Be this as it may, my main problem with Crick and Koch's reasoning is an implicit presupposition that there must be one area where the "final product" comes together. In light of my PMH, I think this a priori assumption is misguided. According to my hypothesis the percept (and conscious states in general) is identical to global processes embedded in feedforward and feedback connections that span over the whole sensorimotor pathway, including the PNS and the CNS. This shows that the above authors' insistence on the percept "not being located at the level of the PNS" is something well taken under my approach, because I also do not think that it is located there. But I part ways with these theorists when they infer that the percept must be somewhere else, namely in some cortical area. I think the percept is the very process itself, and not some final product. I call these views of visual awareness, and consciousness in general, in its relation to the nervous system, "the refinery view," by analogy to an oil refinery plant. Oil refineries are complex systems of pipes and various chemical processing units whose function is to transform crude oil into several petroleum products, like gasoline, kerosene, diesel fuel, asphalt, and many more. The above authors think of the nervous system as such refinery, and of conscious experience as the refined final product of the system. It is as if the brain told you: "Don't worry, I will do all the processing, you just sit back and enjoy the scene!" The assumption of the refinery view is a philosophical one, just like my PMH, so my challenging it in this book is far from misplaced.

By contrast, another group of theories, which I am sympathetic to, are unlike the serialist approaches in that their model of how conscious experience is generated is an integrated system of mutual interactions, both feedforward and feedback, which system at the same time transcends the cortical hierarchies (figure 2.1). These *interactionist* approaches have been proposed by Zeki (1993), Lamme and Roelfsema (2000), and Bullier (2001). These are large-scale neuronal theories of the visual system, according to which feedback connections from higher areas to lower ones play an integral, constitutive part in the percept and the qualities of the percept are reduced to these cross-hierarchical nonserial interactions. As I called the feedforward model "the refinery view," I would call this one, and my own PMH, "the Christmas lights view": it would be crazy to build a lighting system for your Christmas tree such that the electrical impulse travels through a lot of units that manipulate it

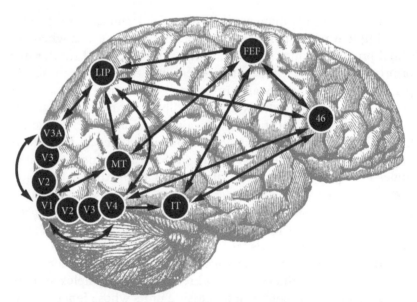

Figure 2.1 Feedback and feedforward connections of the Primary Visual Area (V1) to a subset of other visual areas. (Redrawn from Tong 2003)

only to make a single light bulb or LED light up at the very top of it, while the rest of the tree is in total darkness!

Bullier (2001: 97), for instance, points out that the Marr type feedforward approach is inapplicable to any realistic visual scene. As soon as the scene is noisy, and it is almost always so, due to shadows, occlusions, and various lighting conditions, the feedforward model predicts that the system is unable to identify objects and human figures, because according to the model the processes of segmentation and integration are dissociated. Segmentation takes place early in processing, whereas integration is a higher level phenomenon. Yet, the real human visual system deals very easily with such noisy scenes. There is more empirical evidence for the integrated interactive model, but I won't go into more detail, as I want to move to the topic of causation versus constitution when it comes to the visual percept and its correlated nervous system pathways. Figure 2.1 depicts both the feedforward and feedback connections of V1.

II Causal Versus Constitutive Contribution

As I said, I am sympathetic to interactionism. PMH can be seen as a more extreme version of interactionism, as it extends the integrated basis of sensory consciousness so as to include PNS components (though, as you will see in chapter 6, I do not go as far as to bring consciousness beyond the borders of the nervous system). An influential view in psychology that is congenial to my hypothesis is James Gibson's ecological approach to perception (1966, 1979). One important point that Gibson stresses, which is what my book tries to put to philosophical work, is that there are no privileged levels of the nervous system when it comes to explaining how perception works:

> Instead of postulating that the brain constructs information from the input of a sensory nerve, we can suppose that the centers of the nervous system, including the brain, resonate to information. (Gibson 1966: 267)

> A perceptual system, to repeat, is not composed of an organ and a nerve. The nervous system is part and parcel of any perceptual system, and the centers of the nervous system, from lower to higher, participate in its activity. Organ adjustments are probably controlled by lower centers, selective attention by intermediate centers, and conceptual attention by the highest centers. (Gibson 1966: 271)

The claim of PMH is that PNS processes, when they occur as causal components in a sensory and motor loop, can be considered not as causes of experiences, but as constituent processes of it. However, certainly they are causes and effects of CNS processes. And various components within the CNS are parts of a causal chain too. Because of this causal role, theorists are especially careful when confronted with claims that a certain cortical area "enters consciousness directly." Here is a quote from Tong:

> Lesion studies indicate that V1 is necessary for normal visual function and awareness. After considerable research and debate, early scientists identified V1 as the primary cortical site of vision. Cortical bullet wounds in soldiers revealed a precise retinotopic map in V1, as these small lesions in V1 led to scotomas or phenomenal blindness restricted to corresponding regions of the visual field. *Do these findings indicate that V1 itself is important for visual awareness or that damage to V1 robs higher visual areas of their necessary input?* (2003: 220) (emphasis added)

And the same point stated by Goebel et al.:

> Lesion studies indicate that V1 is necessary for normal visual function and awareness. Small lesions in V1 lead to scotomas or phenomenal blindness restricted to corresponding regions of the visual field as expected from the retinotopic organization of V1....*However, these findings do not answer the question whether V1 itself is important for visual awareness, because the lesions disrupt the flow of information from V1 to higher visual areas.* (2004: 1300) (emphasis added)

The problem seems to be that whatever evidence there is, from lesion or disconnection studies, for potential constitutive contribution of a cortical area to experience, it is also evidence for its merely causal contribution. Indeed, as far as causal sufficiency is concerned current evidence shows that none of the areas involved in the visual system is sufficient:

> According to current evidence from lesion studies, neither activity in V1 nor in higher visual areas is sufficient for awareness. A recent study of blindsight patients has shown that in the absence of V1 visual signals can still reach many extrastriate areas via subcortical projections but that activity in the extrastriate areas seems incapable of generating normal conscious experiences (Goebel *et al.* 2001). It might be that the relationship between activity in certain visual areas and awareness is flexible and situation dependent rather than hard wired. (Goebel et al. 2004: 1300)

There is also a philosophical problem here, as rightly pointed out by Lawrence Shapiro (2010: ch. 6). The problem is that we are dangerously close to, if not in the middle of, a merely verbal dispute about whether some part of the neuro-computational system is characterizeable as a causal contributor, or as a constituent of experience. Suppose that, whenever you claim to have shown that some lower level of the nervous system, or even some PNS component, or even some worldly component is essential or necessary for conscious experience, your opponent claims, as for instance Ned Block does in his review of Alva Noë's (2004) book,[5] that all you managed to show is the causal contribution of that cortical area, or part of the PNS, to experience. Your opponent could also add that your claim amounts to begging the question. The question that arises at this point is: begging the question against whom? Well, it must be against those who claim that what you take as an essential constituent is only a causal component. But those who claim the latter are equally begging the question here. By stating that it is more likely that your alleged constituent is a causal contributor, they actually presuppose that, for some reason, experience is an end product partly caused by your alleged constituent. My point is that we are doomed to begging the question against one another's views. However, given that both my PMH and the opponent's view are philosophical hypotheses, we can beg the question with more or less philosophical benefit; and I claim that I can beg it with a lot more benefit. The rest of the book is dedicated to such "useful question-begging," if you want, or, more precisely, to the new light the PMH throws upon various widely discussed topics in the philosophy of mind (though in chapter 7, where I discuss proprioception, I do propose an argument for the constitutiveness claim).

[5] See Block 2005: 263.

3

Return of the C Fibers; or, Philosophers' Lack of Nerve

"Bernard Williams, a very good English philosopher thought he had a good joke when he said, 'Well, maybe the mind is the brain ... in Australia'"—reports Australian philosopher David Armstrong, in a 2006 interview on ABC Radio National (Australia), on the occasion of celebrating fifty years since the first occurrence in print of the mind-brain identity thesis.[1] Armstrong offers this as a story about how the phrase 'Australian Materialism' with its negative connotations,[2] was introduced to the philosophical vocabulary. There is an English-Australian exchange of ironies here, but maybe the real irony is that from today's perspective Bernard Williams's rhetorical attempt is self-undermining, as we (Australians or not) could equally respond to him: "Well, maybe the mind is not the brain ... in England."

There is a second irony as well. In the same interview, Gerard O'Brien of Adelaide University remarks: "When I got there, there was still this view at Oxford that the Australian Materialism, as it was called by then, was a very naïve position and the attitude was

---

[1] The first published paper arguing for the identity thesis was by Ullin T. Place (1956).

[2] It's not the only time 'Australian ways of doing philosophy' are put under the ironical pens of the 'center'; thus John Heil: "... in the English-speaking world, American anti-realists have descended from the likes of Goodman, Kuhn, and Sellars; in Britain, from Wittgenstein via Dummett. Australia, isolated and out of the loop evolutionarily, continues as a stronghold of realists and marsupials" (Heil 1989: 65).

that it was really only held by colonialists out there in Australia, who really hadn't thought in a very deep way about these ideas." The irony is that the colonialist mentality is rather present in the negative connotations that some English philosophers were suggesting, if O'Brien is right, with the phrase 'Australian Materialism'.

I have mentioned these points not merely as curiosities, to the extent that they are considered so, but as part of the main line of thought in this chapter, the idea that we can gain knowledge about a philosophical conundrum involving debates about 'the right concept C' of some phenomenon P, if we become more open-minded about the possibility of others' concepts of the same phenomenon, and consequently less certain about our own concept C being *the* concept of P. From this general observation, we can then derive various applications to concrete philosophical debates. In this chapter, I'm interested in the problem of consciousness and physicalism. In the first section, I will briefly introduce the case of an African people's, the Akan's conceptual scheme regarding mental phenomena and mental concepts and its implications for the 'physicalism *versus* dualism' debate about phenomenal consciousness. In the second section, I offer a criticism of contemporary philosophy of mind in its neglect of some details of neuroscience that, as I will argue, *do* make a difference to the purely conceptual issues in the physicalism debate, via the "folk neuroscience" that I argue for. In the third section, I present some thought experiments to the conclusion that it makes perfect sense to think of mental properties as physical properties, without the need to posit phenomenal concepts. I explain, in effect, the failure of certain conceivability experiments, once the concepts are reinterpreted. The guiding idea is that once we take the peripheral nervous system seriously and become less fixated on the brain, intuitive-seeming arguments against physicalism become less credible.

I.   *Well, Maybe the Mind Is the Brain ... Somewhere*

Philosophy in the English-speaking world involves, besides the usual logical analysis of arguments, theories, and so on, a lot of appeal to intuition, or what authors try to sell as intuitive understanding of some concept or other. It is partly due to such felicitous matches between what an author takes as intuitive and what his or her readers find so that some ideas become so influential. Names like Gettier, Kripke, Putnam come to one's mind. Things, however, started to

change lately. Although in an inchoate phase at the moment, experimental philosophy shows us an alternative to the blank appeal to
'ordinary intuition' and raises the challenge of actually confirming
the existence of alleged intuitions empirically. Most of this research
is done in the United States, on American-acculturated subjects, but
there are exceptions, when a cross-cultural element plays an important role in the experiments.[3]

The mind-body problem, or the problem of how to understand
mental phenomena within a broadly physicalistic picture of the
world, is one where alleged intuitions and alleged concepts of the
mind find their best soil. Anti-physicalist arguments that appeal to
the notion of phenomenal properties, or qualia, or properties in virtue of which there is something it is like to experience the world,
which are not entailed by the physical facts of the world, are all
based on the phenomenal type of concepts about various mental
phenomena, that we all are supposed to possess, besides other types
of mental concepts (e.g., behavioral-functional). Most physicalists
involved in this debate accept the existence of the phenomenal concept of mind and try to accommodate within a broadly physicalist
ontology the anti-physicalist intuitions that seem to flow from it.
The question, however, is whether, supposing we do possess the
phenomenal conceptualization of the mind, what we take as the
concept of mind is really *the* concept of mind, or *a* concept of
mind.

When it comes to cross-cultural understanding of some ordinary
concepts with potential philosophical import, and especially in the
African studies perspective, I favor what I call 'interactivism', as
opposed to three other approaches that seem to have been in place in
the cultural anthropology with philosophical flavor; in chronologi-
cal order: (i) Eurocentrism (comparativism and evolutionism of a
sort that takes the *others'* concepts as rudimentary, impoverished,
backward); (ii) Cultural relativism (which takes, as Johannes Fabian
([1983] 2002) puts it, other cultures *in* their own terms, but not *on*
their own terms, that is, considers other cultures as fenced off
enclaves, incommensurable with ours, or at least whose worldview
is not to be taken at face value), and (iii) Structural-functionalism

---

[3]Such an attempt is to be found in Mallon, Machery, Nichols, and Stich 2004,
where the authors try to test the Kripkean intuitions against the description theory
of names by appeal to comparative, American-Chinese, study involving university
students as subjects. Most progress in experimental philosophy, however, has been
made in connection to moral intuitions and moral psychology; for an overview and
connections to normative ethics, see Kwame Anthony Appiah 2008.

(which is interested in large patterns across cultures, but neglects differences and local phenomena).

In metaphilosophical context, interactivism about other cultures' concepts or conceptual schemes is the requirement to take these not as curiosities, exotica, and so on, but as actual data to contribute to professional philosophical debates; in other words, interactivism takes both our and other cultures' ordinary concepts at face value when it comes to the point that philosophical argument needs the boost of intuitions. It is, therefore, neither a relativist approach nor a supremacist one, but what I take to be the most reasonable universalism, a philosophical dialogue across cultures, or philosophical cross-cultural understanding.[4]

Such an interactive approach is not widely practiced, but not completely missing either; it is an emergent phenomenon.[5] Ghanian philosopher Kwame Gyekye's book, *An Essay on African Philosophical Thought: The Akan Conceptual Scheme* ([1987] 1995) is an attempt to discuss the Akan people's metaphysical concepts of person, time, causation, mind-body relations, on their own terms. The Akan approach to mind and body is a multifaceted one. Our category of mind *simpliciter* (if there is such), or the category of MIND that makes it synonymous with the concept PERSON, is divided into two categories of substantial mental entity, the *sunsum* and the *okra*. The former is the individual spirit of a person, assumed by anthropologists and sociologists to come from the father at conception and not being divine (Gyekye 1995: 89), and the latter is a sort of life force sent by the high god, Nyame, and departs the person's body at the person's last breath (Appiah 2004: 27), although Gyekye does not exclude that *sunsum* and *okra* might in the end refer to a single basic immaterial soul-like substance (Gyekye 1995:47, 95). It

[4] When it comes to the question of African philosophy, especially the question of what metaphilosophical theoretical attitude one should have vis-à-vis the oral, preliterate African thought, four broad approaches have been identified (Birt 1991): (a) Ethnophilosophy (the view that the oral tradition has to be taken as the philosophical tradition in Africa, even though it is not systematic and it involves religious/mythological elements); (b) Sage philosophy (a focus on particular persons considered wise during history, equating philosophy with the sayings of these); (c) Ideological philosophy (equating philosophy with the ideas put forward by ideologues of the postcolonial Socialist-Nationalist movements); and (d) Professional philosophy (that is, denying any African philosophical tradition as such, except in the postcolonial period, when professionally trained, systematic philosophers emerge). Interactivism would be a fifth position, partly combining positions (a) and (d), but going well beyond a simple such combination, by taking ethnophilosophical ideas and concepts as input for systematic philosophizing in the style of the professional approach.

[5] For a model, see Appiah 2004.

is *sunsum* that is the seat and capacity of thinking (Gyekye 1995: 63), so it is similar to a Cartesian concept of a mind or person. We can say, synthesizing and simplifying, that the Akan are a sort of substance dualists when it comes to persons.

The body, *nipadua*, is also part of the concept of a person. What is most interesting, the mentalistic language that sometimes guides our intuitions about distinguishing mental from bodily attributes is completely missing in Akan language, for the corresponding concepts in English. Gyekye offers a long enough list of mentalistic terms in English, translated into Akan, then retranslated etymologically into English expressions (pp. 166–68). He remarks:

> The English language, brimful of mentalistic expressions, has misled thinkers into an ontology of the mental.... It can be seen that the mentalistic (English) expressions ... translated into Akan actually become physicalistic expressions. In Akan, that is, the mentalistic expressions in English actually refer to the body or some organs of the body such as the eyes, chest, stomach, heart, ears, head, etc., but the words of the original sentences in English made no reference to parts of the body. (p. 165)

Some examples of what Gyekye is talking about are shown in table 3.1.

The emphasized lexical parts in Akan correspond to the emphasized words in English denoting body parts. All these sentences and expressions in Akan are used literally.

Again, synthesizing and simplifying, we might say: the Akan, while substance dualist about persons, are property physicalists about the mind; more exactly, when it comes to mental properties, they are logical behaviorists.

Table 3.1 Akan behavioristic mental concepts (following Gyekye 1995: 166–68)

English ...	into Akan ...	and etymologically into English
1. I am happy	*M'ani agye*	'My *eyes* are brightened'
2. I am in despair	Mehome te me ho	'My *breath* is breaking apart'
3. I am aware	M'ani da meho so	'My *eyes* are on my body'
4. Awareness/ consciousness	*ani*daho	'One's *eyes* are widely open'
5. Peace of mind	Asomdwee	'Coolness/calmness of the *ear*'
6. Grief/sorrow	Awerehow	Reference is made to the heart
7. Apprehension	Ayamhyehye	'One's *stomach* burns'

What are we to make of such a situation, even if, I'm sure, it is presumably not the whole story? In light of the success that property dualist arguments by Saul Kripke (1972), Thomas Nagel (1974), Frank Jackson (1982), and David Chalmers (1996) achieved these years, in the sense that nowadays the qualia-based, phenomenal concept involving conceivability intuitions against physicalism are broadly taken as evidence to be accounted for by physicalists, one option is to adopt relativism. One would then say that these arguments work within 'our culture', but they are powerless within 'other cultures'. I don't know whether any of these arguments have actually been translated into, say, Ghanian language, but one might raise doubts as to whether the power those intuitions proved to have over Western readers would carry over to Ghanian readers. However, instead of carrying forward such speculation, it is worth noting one important point, namely, that there is both a dependence of conceivability intuitions on the concepts that are involved, and one between the concepts involved and the more general conceptual scheme within which they are embedded, and which might vary from culture to culture, or from time to time.

This, however, does not mean that we *must* go relativist and make the facile move against the property dualist arguments and intuitions, claiming that they merely show the truth of a pair of conditionals, like: 'if one possesses phenomenal concepts, one can conceive of zombies (physical duplicates of conscious being lacking consciousness whatsoever)' and 'if one does not possess phenomenal concepts, one cannot conceive of zombies'. This claim I find too weak. Failing to possess a concept is not merely an empirical matter; there is a normative element to it as well. Second, concepts are not fixed and unchanging. The real lesson is to realize that we can reflect on our own concepts, just like the Akan could reflect on theirs, and this is especially true when it comes to philosophical analysis of these concepts. One can summarize it this way:

> In the long run, it will turn out, I'm sure, that people will decide there is no *sunsum*; but I'm equally convinced that eventually we shall lose our belief in the *mind*. (Appiah 2004: 33) (emphasis in original)

I will now turn to the issue of trying to bend *our* allegedly phenomenal concept of the mind or mental phenomena. Even if the Akan behavioristic language might be too far apart from what we can do with our concepts, I will argue that some folk-neuroscientific reevaluation is possible and plausible, and it will make the mind-brain

identity thesis, or something in that spirit, coherent, and the phenomenal concept based intuitions much weaker.

II. Folk Neuroscience and the Philosophy of Mind

Philosophers who care about conceptual issues usually don't care
about empirical details. In the philosophy of mind one comes across
the formula 'in principle, mental states are reducible to brain states;
the details don't matter'. Functionalism, both in its analytic and in
its empirical version, asserts that whatever, say, the pain state will
turn out to be, it will be a functional property, roughly a state that is
caused by some pain-specific stimuli and causing, together with
other functional states, pain-specific behavior; again, details, neurophysiological or cognitive-architectural, don't matter, as far as the
philosophical problem is concerned.

The early mind-brain identity thesis (Place 1956; Feigl 1958;
Smart 1959) was soon augmented with a functionalist component
(Lewis 1966; Armstrong 1968) and came to be known as Central
State Materialism. The motivation for the name was given by the
fact that now the identity thesis was more specific, identifying mental states with states of the Central Nervous System (CNS), by which
philosophers just meant 'state of the cortex'. Details were not important, only for the main idea to be coherent.

For some reason or other, the same philosophers have widely
started using the alleged identity statement 'pain = C fibers firing' as
their paragon example of what the identity thesis is all about, what
the Central State Materialist is committed to, and consequently of
what the opponents of the thesis are supposed to deal with if they
are to falsify the thesis.

The case of 'pain = C fibers firing' is what I call an instance of
folk neuroscience, which philosophers are happy to practice, disre-
garding the details. Folk neuroscience is not in itself bad; actually,
what I will do in the next section is such an exercise in folk neuroscience, meant to boost the intuitions in favor of the identity thesis
in some form. However, in this specific case, 'pain = C fibers firing',
philosophers' folk-neuroscientific sketchiness and neglect of details
amounts to a blunder. C fibers have nothing to do with the CNS;
they are nerve fibers to be found in the PNS. They are one of the
two nociceptive (responding to noxious stimuli) types of nerves.
They don't even directly project to the cortex, but to the spinal
cord; yet, philosophers had no qualms in calling C fiber states 'brain
states'.

Of course, I'm not saying that any one philosopher was seriously thinking that 'pain = C fibers firing' is a true candidate for a piece of what the identity thesis implies; many were explicit in stating something like 'well, because exact details don't matter, let's use such an example'. I certainly never took this example seriously.[6] What I'm saying is that this statement could not even be used as acceptable *folk* neuroscience, and that it is ironic that what they called 'Central State Materialism' had actually nothing to do with central states, but with peripheral ones.

However, the real irony is that, if what I am going to argue here is plausible, they were basically right: pain is C fiber firing and anything else that involves the PNS's activity within pain states! They were right for the wrong reasons.

Let's start with filling in some minimal genuine neuroscientific detail into the 'C fiber picture' of my folk neuroscience of pain. The *Gate Control Theory of Pain* (GCT), elaborated by Ronald Melzack and Patrick D. Wall in the 1960s[7] is a true success story of theoretical neurophysiology. Its influence has been enormous, it has been confirmed in both animal and human subjects, and, as a result, there has not been any need to elaborate a newer theory of the neurological mechanisms of pain (Fitzgerald 2010). In order to appreciate its force, it is worth describing how it superseded its two earlier rivals: the *Specificity Theory* (ST) and the *Pattern Theory* (PT).

ST assumes that there are nerve endings in body tissue, specialized as 'pain receptors', which project to a 'pain center' in the brain. The receptors transmit the nerve impulse via the A-delta fibers and C fibers of the PNS. A-delta fibers are thick, have a fast conduction speed of nerve impulses, and a low threshold of activation; they are responsible for the first stage, sharp pain sensation occurring immediately after tissue injury. C fibers, on the other hand, are thin, have a slow conduction speed, and a high threshold of activation; they are responsible for the dull, long, constant pain sensation whose onset occurs in a second stage after injury. As Melzack and Wall note (1965: 971), ST's strength is the part about the specialized nerves in the PNS, that is, that they are specialized in responding to noxious stimuli (hence they are called 'nociceptive'), the A-delta and C fibers. Its weakness, however, is an implicit conceptual connection that is

[6]Roland Puccetti (1977), who is the first to point out the C-fiber blunder in print, seems to have taken them seriously, at least as I read him.

[7]See Melzack and Wall 1965.

posited—by the use of the terms 'pain receptors in the body tissue' and 'pain center in the brain'—between the feeling of pain and the noxious peripheral stimulation and a supposed center of pain in the brain, where the seat of the feeling of pain is supposed to be. This implies an implicit model of direct-communication line system between the skin and the brain, which runs against clinical evidence:

> The pathological pain states of causalgia (a severe burning pain that may result from a partial lesion of a peripheral nerve), phantom limb pain (which may occur after amputation of a limb), and the peripheral neuralgias (which may occur after peripheral nerve infections or degenerative diseases) provide a dramatic refutation of the concept of a fixed, direct-line nervous system. (Melzack and Wall 1965: 971)

There is also psychological and physiological evidence that fails to support this view, but we won't have time here to enter the details.

The main rival of this theory was PT, which recognizes that various activities in the CNS may intervene between the stimulus and the pain sensation, which may invalidate any notion of 'psycho-physical law' holding between the intensity of stimulus in the PNS and intensity of the felt sensation. PT proposes two mechanisms to account for the evidence regarding pain: a mechanism of spatially and temporally patterned activity of nonspecific, nonspecialized fibers at the level of PNS, and a CNS mechanism of central summation which would account, for example, for amplification of stimuli of low intensity coming from damaged peripheral nerves. PT is a group of theories, some of which stress the PNS component, others the CNS component of the pain generation mechanism. PT does not run into troubles of the kind mentioned in connection with ST, but the various theories failed to be unified and experimentally confirmed.

Finally, GCT is a theory that is considered as best integrating positive aspects of ST and PT, as well as novel in proposing a single complex mechanism that accounts for all the evidence, psychological, physiological, clinical, and experimental. The basic idea of GCT is that there is a gate control mechanism in the *substantia gelatinosa* (in the spinal cord), which modulates the synaptic transmission (intensity and other characteristics of the nerve impulse) coming from the peripheral nerves (A-delta and C fibers of the PNS). The mechanism of gate control determines the quality of felt pain as a function of three stimulus specific parameters: the ongoing activity in the CNS which precedes the stimulus, the stimulus-evoked activity, and the relative balance of large versus small fibers (A-delta versus C fibers). Moreover, GCT also involves the existence of an efferent (downwards conducting) brain trigger mechanism that modulates afferent (upward conducting) nerve impulse from the PNS, whose influences are also mediated through the gate control system. The theory explains clinical data such as hyperalgesia in peripheral neuropathy, phantom limb pain, and spontaneous pain (unrelated to tissue damage). The basic mechanism that explains these phenomena is the gate system failing to inhibit (i.e., gates are open) the nerve impulse when it is weak as it arrives from damaged nerve bundles (damaged A-delta fibers in the case of neuropathy-related hyperalgesia), from peripheral regions unrelated to where the damage is felt as having occurred (in the case of phantom limb pain), and from random low-level ongoing activity in the PNS (in the case of spontaneous pain). The efferent central mechanism that I have mentioned accounts for the great variability of pain among subjects, even in the case of severe lesions. Finally, there is a whole literature on therapeutic applications of GCT, but this much will suffice for our exercise in folk neuroscience that is to follow.

What are we to make of all these facts? The main point of expounding this theory of pain mechanisms is to prepare the ground for a couple of folk-neuroscientific ideas that can have an effect, at a purely conceptual level, on ongoing philosophical debates. The first such idea is that, contrary to the superficial way we, philosophers, tend to handle scientific data when it comes to the physicalism debate, or the identity thesis, let us first admit that the property of *being in pain* is not a very subtle and discerning notion. Relatedly, a sentence like 'pain = C fibers firing' embodies certain assumptions that are simply nonsensical once the neuroscientific theory and evidence are brought in. Indeed, the very notion of a 'pain center' that philosophers of mind tend to simply assume, serving as a neural correlate of pain, and as a terminus region of the nervous system where the felt sensation finally emerges, is, as pointed out by Melzack and Wall (1965: 976), nonsense in the context of actual data from neuroscience:

> The concept of a "pain center" in the brain is totally inadequate to account for the sequences of behavior and experience. Indeed, the concept is pure fiction, unless virtually the whole brain is considered to be the "pain center," because the thalamus, the limbic system, the hypothalamus, the brain-stem reticular formation, the parietal cortex, and

the frontal cortex are all implicated in pain perception.... The idea of a "terminal center" in the brain which is exclusively responsible for pain sensation and response therefore becomes meaningless.[8]

This point is very important in the context of philosophical talk about neural correlates consciousness, when philosophers tend to think of these as brain regions or centers. Similarly, philosophers talk about 'realizers of mental states', and what they mean is, again some brain region that is active. How we should instead think of the neural underpinning of mental phenomena, like pain, is by way of complex interactive mechanisms generating feedforward and feedback processes involving not only the brain, but the peripheral nerves and the spinal cord too.

Why is this important, as far as philosophy is concerned? It is important because some of our mental concepts might change as a result of thinking in terms of an adequate folk neuroscience when it comes to analyzing the mind-body problem. I offer such an attempt at conceptual change in the remaining two sections.

This brings me to the second folk-neuroscientific idea to extract from the above discussion. Ordinary people's phenomenologically self-evident notion of pain is that it is located in some distal part of the body, not in the brain. Some philosophers, on the other hand, assume that this is an unreflective and uninformed view, either because according to neuroscientific theorizing pain is really in the brain (qualia theory of pain combined with correlation between qualia and brain states), or because pain is an intentional property such that felt location is part of its intentional content (intentionalism about pain), but the property itself is instantiated by the brain. When I cut my finger, I feel the pain in my finger, or I feel the pain of the finger, so I believe that it is located in the finger; yet, philosophers seem to assume, that is a false belief—*always*. It is worth exemplifying this with a quote, say, from an intentionalist about pain, like Michael Tye:

> Token experiences, including pains, are themselves located in the brain. So, there really are no pains inside legs. So, the above experience, in

---

[8] The above folk-neuroscientific fallacy that philosophers tend to commit is akin to what Daniel Dennet identified at the level of psychological concepts as a fallacy that philosophers tend to commit, the so-called Cartesian Theater concept of consciousness—"the view that there is a crucial finish line or boundary somewhere in the brain, marking a place where the order of arrival equals the order of 'presentation' in experience because what happens there is what you are conscious of" (Dennett 1991: 107).

representing that something in the leg is painful, must be misrepresent-
ing what is going on. And this is highly counter-intuitive. Surely, a
person who feels a pain in the leg, in normal circumstances, is not subject to an illusion.

This objection contains a non-sequitur. From the fact that there are
no pains in legs it does not follow that a pain which represents that
some disturbance in a leg is painful is a misrepresentation. When it is
said that a cut in a finger or a burn or a bruise is painful or hurts, what
is meant is (roughly) that it is *causing* a feeling, namely the very feeling
the person is undergoing. (Tye 1995: 228) (emphasis in original)

This idea that the 'feeling of pain' is actually merely *caused* by the
activity of the PNS is widely assumed by philosophers of mind,
especially by the very popular causal-role functionalist theory, and
it is an instance of the bad folk neuroscience we have been
discussing.

But if we take the above neuroscientific ideas seriously, it is
clear, first, that the very idea of the pain, the property, being instantiated at a particular region of the nervous system does not arise,
and, second, ordinary people are, in a sense, right: in this particular
case, when I cut my finger, pain, if we are to talk in terms of location, is partly 'in my finger', as it is some damage to the PNS that
plays an integral role in the whole feedforward and feedback mechanism and process that deserves the name 'pain'.

III.   *Nervous Systems and Closet* Sunsum *Theory*

Here are some linguistic revisions that are prompted by the discussion so far. 'Central State Materialism' should really be replaced
with '*Central-cum-Peripheral* Materialism'; 'Mind-Brain Identity
Thesis' should become 'Mind-[Nervous System] Identity Thesis';
and 'Causal Role Functionalism' should perhaps become 'Global
Synaptic Pattern Functionalism'—the difference here being that the
old folk theory of causal role functionalism implicitly assumes that,
for example, the pain state is a CNS state, by which they mean a
brain state, typically *caused by* noxious stimuli *and the nerve
impulse traveling through the PNS* (though hardly anyone cares to
make this explicit) and *causing* some type of avoidance behavior,
part of the notion of behavior being the activity of the efferent nerve
firings (though, again, hardly anyone cares to make this explicit),
whereas the new folk theory says that pain is a complex feedforward
and feedback process of the relevant integrated CNS *and* PNS synaptic routes.

Let's then turn to some anti-physicalist intuitions that philosophers claim to have. The zombie is a creature conceived as a physical duplicate of an actual conscious being, but lacking consciousness whatsoever. Virtually everyone in the debate agrees that there is an intuition to the effect that such a creature is conceivable. Such conceivability intuitions are then taken for granted and any theory of the mind has to explain them, or explain them away. This is then the problem physicalists have with phenomenal properties, or rather with the phenomenal type of mental concepts. Is it that we first have such phenomenal concepts of pain, anger, pleasure, consciousness, and so on, and because we have them, we can conceive of zombies? Or is it that we can just primitively conceive of zombies, hence we deduce that there is a phenomenal concept of mind that we are committed to? I think there is no explanatory priority either from concepts to conceivability or vice versa; rather, to allude to a formula by Hilary Putnam,[9] concept and conceiving jointly make up concept and conceiving.

However, consider someone, John, who is undergoing pain in the actual world, and the following statements:

(1) Actually, John is in pain.
(2) It is conceivable that there be a physical duplicate of John, John*, who is not in pain.

This is an instance of the zombie intuition. If we unpack the statements so as to involve reference to the nervous system, we get something along the following lines:

(3) Actually, John's nervous system is in a state S, and John is in pain.
(4) It is conceivable that there be a physical duplicate of John's nervous system, S*, such that John's physical duplicate, John*, is not in pain.

With this unpacking, the zombie intuition is still apparently vindicated, but on pain of talking about two types of entities that are subjects of property instantiations: S and S*, on the one hand, instantiating neural properties, and John and John*, on the other, instantiating phenomenal pain.

If we are to keep faithful to our new folk neuroscience, according to which it is nervous systems that are the entities that instantiate

---

[9]Thus Putnam: "If one is to use metaphorical language then let the metaphor be this: the mind and the world jointly make up the mind and the world" (1981: xi).

pain, we should check whether the zombie intuition is still vindicated under such a conceptual scheme. I think it is not:

(5) Actually, nervous system S is in pain.
(6) It is conceivable that there be a physical duplicate of S, S*, such
    that it is not in pain.

I myself think that (6) is plainly false, but you might think otherwise. Still, you have to admit that there is at least a *difference*
between (3)/(4) and (5)/(6)—it is harder to conceive of zombies when
the subject that is assumed to actually instantiate the pain is a nervous system than when it is a person, or phenomenal subject, or
mind.

To further boost this intuition, recall that according to our new
folk neuroscience PNS processes are an integral part of pain. Consider a subject who has suffered peripheral nerve damage, more
exactly, chemical toxicity induced partial destruction of A-delta
fibers, leaving most of the C fibers intact. The subject suffers from
hyperalgesia, (e.g., perceives a soft touch of the skin as pain), as a
result of the damage, which is accounted for by (i) the activity of the
C fibers and (ii) the summation effects that the gate control system
of the *substantia gelatinosa* of the spinal cord and the efferent brain
fibers are responsible for. Suppose the subject is gently touched on
the foot, and the whole pain process starts as a result. We can say:

(7) Actually, the foot is in pain.

But is it intuitive that a zombie foot is conceivable? Consider:

(8) It is conceivable that there be an intrinsic and extrinsic neural
    duplicate of the foot such that it is not in pain.

If zombie feet are not conceivable, on the condition that to attribute
instantiation of pain partly by the foot is correct, then we can move
forward on the afferent neural paths involved in the process of hyperalgesia, from the PNS to the spinal cord, then to the brain stem,
thalamus, cortex, and argue that there is no intuition of zombie versions of these.

It can be objected at this point that our folk neuroscience is
wrong, and that it is not correct to attribute *phenomenal* pain to
nervous systems. But the basis of such an assertion could only be a
closet *sunsum* theory, according to which there are phenomenal
subjects and *they* are supposed to be in pain, not neural subjects,
that is, nervous systems. I suspect that it is this implicit commitment, as well as the 'pain center in the brain' commitment (which

involves an experiencing center), that are responsible for the widely held belief among philosophers that the zombie is intuitive.

I'm not saying that *sunsum* theory is wrong in itself; only that philosophers of mind ought to admit that they are committed to it when pushing the zombie intuition. The Akan *sunsum* concept is, in fact, less pervasive in *their* concept of a mind, as we saw when discussing their behavioristic language when it comes to mental states. On the other hand, the dualists who are pushing the zombie intuition are property dualists, who pride themselves in not being committed to phenomenal substances, things. They should be happy with the formula: 'phenomenal pain is a property of the nervous system'. Yet, such a formula ultimately weakens the zombie intuition considerably.

To substantiate my claim that there is a closet *sunsum* theory held among property dualists, I will quote a couple of passages from David Chalmers's rightly celebrated book, *The Conscious Mind* (1996), where he tries to introduce the zombie idea in an informal way, in which quotes I highlight that in connection with the zombie, whenever it comes to the part about the absence of consciousness, it is the *sunsum* of Chalmers himself that gets involved by implicit reference. Here are the quotes:

> So let us consider *my* zombie twin. This creature is molecule for molecule identical to *me*, and identical in all low-level properties postulated by a complete physics, but he lacks conscious experience entirely. (Some might prefer to call the zombie "it," but I use the personal pronoun; I have grown quite fond of *my* zombie twin.) (Chalmers 1996: 94) (emphasis added)

The innocence of the humorous statement about the use of the personal pronoun "he" for the zombie, instead of the impersonal "it," as a sign of appreciation for the zombie, is lost once we realize that Chalmers could just as well have used an impersonal way of referring *to himself* in this passage, as a result of the intuitiveness of referring to the zombie in an impersonal way. Let us actually replace the personal with the impersonal terms and adjust some sentences for the relevant changes in meaning; we get something less convincing as far as the zombie idea is concerned:

> So let us consider nervous system S's (N.B. Chalmers's nervous system) zombie twin, S^*. S^* is molecule for molecule identical to S, and identical in all low-level properties postulated by a complete physics, but it lacks conscious experience entirely. (Some might prefer to call S "me," but I use the impersonal pronoun; I have grown quite less fond of *myself*.)

The second quote is the following:

> A zombie is just something physically identical to *me*, but *which* has no conscious experience—all is dark *inside*. (Chalmers 1996: 96) (emphasis added)

Besides the contrast between "me" and "which" (not "who") that reflects the difference between a person and a zombie, the metaphor 'dark inside' strikes me as out of place when we replace the person Chalmers with the nervous system:

> A zombie is just something physically identical to nervous system *S*, but which has no conscious experience—all is dark *inside*.

Inside what? It must be inside nervous system S^*, the physical duplicate of nervous system *S*. But how could we make sense of the metaphorical dark *versus* light in the case of a nervous system? It can't be that dark alludes to lack of activity inside the system or the fibers—there is a lot excitation (or excitation-inhibition cycles) going on in both systems. It also can't be that there is a mental subject, an entity who experiences these excitations inside; that would, or ought to be, an embarrassment for the property dualist, whose official commitment is to brains *qua brains*—or, given our argument, nervous systems *qua nervous systems*—instantiating phenomenal pain.

Those who think that zombies are conceivable, might insist that even though our folk neuroscience brings about the right verdicts about the notion of pain as such, still, there is also *phenomenal* pain, which we fail to account for. So even though a nervous system *S*, undergoing the relevant nerve impulse transmission processes, but without the system being in pain is inconceivable, it is still conceivable that the system is not in *phenomenal* pain or that it does not involve the *phenomenal* feel of pain. This idea is bizarre enough. It would entail that there is a notion of 'pain' that has nothing to do with ordinary pain. Since it is accepted that the nervous system undergoing a certain nervous process without it being in pain is inconceivable, it follows that ordinary pain logically supervenes on processes of the nervous system. On the other hand, 'phenomenal pain' putatively fails to logically supervene on such nervous system processes. What follows is that phenomenal pain fails to supervene on pain. But then it what sense is it really *pain*? Isn't it more plausible to simply abandon such phenomenal concepts, in light of the correct folk neuroscience and the intuitions that it supports, and admit that they are empty?

In earlier work (Aranyosi 2010, 2011), I put forward two distinct arguments against the conceivability of zombies, which I still believe to be effective, and which did not attack the very idea of the legitimacy of phenomenal concepts whenever one is talking about conscious states.[10] However, here I have tried to weaken the case for taking the phenomenal concepts as given and immutable. Of course, phenomenology is important, and, as it will become apparent later, I myself am heavily relying on it in my arguments. At the same time, when moving to the neuroscientific level of discourse, where the focus is not the person as such, but the nervous system, including the peripheral parts of it, I think the epistemic intuitions of the zombie type should come out as considerably weakened. Recall from the introductory chapter that conscious states are best thought of as distributional properties of the nervous system, encompassing both central and peripheral structures. If this is so, then at the peripheral levels, like the level of an individual sensory fiber, we can legitimately talk about and ask whether that fiber is conscious or not. This will probably sound puzzling for many, so let me explain it.[11]

The fiber can be considered conscious in the sense of its activity being constitutive of a conscious state, say, a sensory state. What "conscious" means at that level is, of course, nothing but being active or firing in a certain way, the way depending on what global conscious state it is part of. In a manner reminiscent of the Estonian biologist Jakob von Uexküll's biosemiotic preoccupations (Uexküll [1934] 2010),[12] let me use the following analogy. Consider the state of being scared. Most ordinarily, we think this is partly a phenomenal state; there is something it is like to be scared. Now consider a dog or a cat. Do we attribute the state of being scared to

---

[10]The so-called "phenomenal concepts strategy" (Stoljar 2005) has quickly become the most popular response to the conceivability arguments against physicalism, judging by the sheer number of authors who appear to champion it (e.g., Balog 1999, 2009, 2012; Diaz-Leon 2008, 2010; Loar 1997; Papineau 2002, 2007; Schroer 2010; Tye 1999).

[11]An anonymous referee was dissatisfied with, or puzzled by, the very idea of a fiber being conscious.

[12]Uexküll was interested in animals as subjects interacting with their environment, and his work was the first to deal with very simple, and for that reason "noncanonical" and marginalized animals like ticks, sea-urchins, amoebae, sea worms, etc., as subjects rather than as objects of study, like in physiology (in Uexküll's words, as machine operators rather than as machines). His original ideas were acknowledged by many philosophers, including Heidegger, Merleau-Ponty, and Deleuze, but were popularized by Hungarian semiotician Thomas Sebeok in guise of the new field of biosemiotics. See Sebeok 2001 for a history of biosemiotics.

such creatures? I think we do it ordinarily and seemingly straight-forwardly, even though, as I see it at least, the way it is like for a dog to be scared must be very different from the way it is like for us to be scared. So "being scared" as applied to the dog refers to a *doggy-scare* and is attributed via the behavioral patterns exhibited by the dog in various stimulus contexts. Now consider the sea urchin that Uexküll was interested in. The sea urchin is a globular and spiny creature of the ocean, of the genus *Echinometra*, having a relatively simple, brainless nervous system, with three senses: for touch, light, and chemicals, respectively. Sea urchins do not have eyes, but rather their entire body acts like a composite eye (Yerra-milli and Johnsen 2010) in that it is photosensitive and has the role mainly of photically detecting the presence of predators, by the shadow cast by them. When any large enough opaque object approaches, the sea urchin extends its spines in the direction of the stimulus, as a defense reflex. When the big fish approaches, is the normally functioning sea urchin scared? Although we might be reluctant to attribute this state to the sea urchin, by analogy with the fact that when we did attribute it to the dog it was, in fact, in the form of doggy-scare, we could think of a type of "scare" or "anx-iety" that would apply to such simple subjects and call it *sea-urchiny-scare*. This is not to anthropomorphize the sea urchin—it wasn't when we attributed anxiety to the dog. On the contrary, it is to *de-anthropomorphize* it all the way and across all species, *our-selves included* (in our case it would be more appropriate to say "de-personalize"). It is this way that I think about the fiber being conscious, as *fibery-consciousness*. But, I argue, we only get essen-tially the same fiber-consciousness at any level of the nervous system.

The most intuitive way, therefore, in which the fiber could be considered conscious is by its being active, that is, if it fires. To add a further phenomenal layer to the fiber and ask whether it is instan-tiated in all logically possible circumstances in which the conduc-tion properties of the fiber are is not only uneconomical, at this level of simplicity, but, I would venture, even a priori or semanti-cally inadequate. Phenomenal consciousness, appealing to Thomas Nagel's (1974) celebrated formula, is intuitively grasped when we try to think of *what it is like* to experience. But the formula "what it is like to experience" is only proper to be ascribed to whole expe-riencers, that is, to whole persons. Now, at the level of our individ-ual fiber that is firing, unless PMH is an absurd hypothesis (which I obviously think it is not), we can talk of consciousness, or part of what constitutes it, without inadequacy, on the model of distributional properties. To use an analogy, consider a painting depicting a human face. The property *depicting a human face* is a distributional property, where what is distributed is paint over the canvass. Now, we can say that the color patches depicting the nose of the human face constitutively contribute to the distributional property *depicting a human face*, so that for that smaller part of the canvas to be a part of a human face depiction is for it to be colored in a certain way. In the same way, for a fiber to be constitutive part of consciousness, or to be conscious-in-its-own-way in the globally conscious field of the nervous system, is for that fiber to fire in certain ways.

Yet, the notion of what it is like does not apply at this level. But if it does not apply at this level of the nervous system, then by what reason should it apply at higher, brain-based levels of it? If for the fiber to be "conscious" (*in its own way*) is, or even *means*, for it to have a manner of firing, then a "zombie fiber" is inconceivable.[13] And then a zombie foot is inconceivable too; and so is a zombie nervous system. So, when we move to the neuroscientific discourse about consciousness, I argue, we should abandon this phenomenal way of thinking about consciousness.[14]

---

[13] Michael Pelczar and Ben Blumson both objected in connection with an earlier draft that their intuition is (what they consider as) the opposite: the more complex the behavior exhibited by an organism, the less conceivable a zombie version of that organism. For instance, a normal human, talking, reacting to stimuli, expressing herself verbally, etc. is harder to hypothesize to be zombie, than it is to do so in the case of a worm. But I do not claim that it is not harder to imagine that there is nothing it is like to be a human than that there is nothing it is like to be a worm. My point is different. It is that at a suitably simple level of the nervous system we can both (a) talk about consciousness or constitutive contribution to consciousness, and (b) at that level, the notion of what it is like is inadequate. What is adequate, however, is electrical activity. Finally, from that simple level we can move upward to any level of the nervous system and establish that the phenomenal "what it is likeness" is not adequate when talking about consciousness of a nervous system; it is only adequate when we talk at the personal, subjective level of an experiencer. I am grateful to Michael and Ben for pushing me on this issue.

[14] Again, an anonymous referee is dissatisfied with this argument, considering that it might involve a fallacy of the form "if it doesn't apply to the part, it doesn't apply to the whole." But my argument is not based on such a fallacy; what it says is rather "because there is no essential difference, as far as electrical activity is concerned, between single neuron and a higher level of organization of many neurons, if it is (a) adequate to talk about consciousness at the single neuron's level understanding it as electrical activity, and (b) inadequate to talk about "what it is like" at that level, then (c) it is also inadequate to talk about "what it is like" at any higher level of organization of active neurons.

Let me briefly touch upon another anti-physicalist argument, which some people take as even more intuitive than the zombie intuition: the knowledge argument proposed by Frank Jackson (1982). Jackson's character, Mary, is assumed to be a person who has been confined to a black-and-white environment, has never experienced any colors, and has acquired complete cognitive-neuroscientific knowledge of human vision, including color vision. If physicalism is true, the argument goes, there is nothing to learn, no piece of new knowledge about human color experiences to be acquired by Mary, since Mary knows all matters physical regarding the human visual system. Yet, it is intuitive or obvious that when Mary is released from her colorless environment and sees a red rose for the first time she *does* acquire a new piece of knowledge, about human color experiences, she comes to know what it is like to experience red. Hence, physicalism is false.

The literature on the knowledge argument has by now grown massive, and it is not my goal here to review the responses that have been put forward, but rather to propose a new line of attack based on what we have been arguing so far. The first thing to note is that, *strictly speaking*, at the exact time when Mary sees the red rose for the first time she is actually suffering *loss* of some knowledge—the visually based neuroscientific knowledge about her own experience of the red rose, which she can't have while experiencing the red rose. However, this does not really affect the initial assumption of complete neuroscientific knowledge, as she could acquire this piece of knowledge later, when checking the visual data that the scanning devices have been transmitting to her computer while she was experiencing the rose.

However, let's try to think of Mary as a nervous system, and her states of knowledge as states of that nervous system.[15] Let's call

---

[15] This move has been questioned by some people who read the manuscript, including one anonymous referee, the idea being that it is not legitimate to talk in terms of nervous systems as "knowing" or "believing." For instance, the referee asked: "Would we say that I'm conscious of the chair in front of me, but at the same time my nervous system is conscious of the activations that underpin A?" There is a misunderstanding here and a double standard on the part of the same people who are happy to reject the substance dualist doctrine of a self that is distinct from the body or organism. The sense in which I use phrases like "Nervous system M comes to know that P" is simply the sense in which one should have no trouble paraphrasing "John comes to know that P" as "This organism comes to know that P." My point is simply that if you are not fond of the doctrine of a Cartesian soul, you should have no qualms in applying to nervous systems as subjects whatever predicate (epistemic, doxastic, deontic, etc.) applies to persons as subjects.

Mary's nervous system M. Knowledge that p can roughly be glossed as true and reliably generated belief that p. Now the argument would look something like this:

(9) In the black-and-white environment, nervous system M has all the reliably generated true beliefs about the neurophysiological aspects of color vision.

(10) When experiencing a red rose for the first time, M acquires new reliably generated *true* beliefs about color vision (i.e., comes to know what it is like to experience red).

(11) Therefore, there are truths about color vision which are not neurophysiological truths.

The problem is that (10) reads too much into the situation. One thing that is obviously true about system M when confronted with the red rose is that M has now several of its components activated by visual stimuli: the retina, the optic nerve fibers, the CNS components involved in visual processing. And activation of the relevant paths for the first time *just is* nervous system M experiencing red for the first time. Nervous system M's coming to know what it is like to experience red *just is* M's coming to experience red (i.e., get activated in the relevant parts)—zombie optic nerves are as inconceivable as zombie feet. To think otherwise, that is, to think that there is more either to system M experiencing red or to system M coming to know what its own activation is like, is, again, to be committed to *sunsum* theory, to system M containing some phenomenal mind 'inside' itself.

Second, knowledge implies belief. But what is the belief component of the so-called 'knowing what it is like'? Believing what it is like? It does not make much sense. It must then be, on the model of other cases of beliefs implied by cases of knowing-*wh* attributions,[16] believing *that* it is like ... Like what? Well, it will be agreed that the "like" here is not comparative; it is not as in cases when we say "experiencing red is like experiencing pink." This is so, among other reasons, because Mary would come to know what it is like to see red even if she has no idea what experiencing pink is like. What we are left with is *apparently* Mary believing *that* it is like *this* to see red, but in reality we are left with just Mary believing *this*, where "this" refers to the very experience of red. The reason is that Mary might not even have the concept of RED at all, but would still come to

---

[16]For example, knowing what John said implies believing that what he said was P, or knowing when the party starts implies believing that it starts at t.

allegedly "believe that it is like *this* to see red," which just means that she has some doxastic attitude to the experience itself, without any thought involving the concept RED.

What could it then possibly mean "to believe *this*"? If taken as occurrent, then the alleged belief is problematic because it only needs the occurrence of the experience in order for it to occur. The closest we can get to such a case are introspective beliefs, which I am aware that most philosophers who wrote on the knowledge argument do consider Mary's knowledge to be based on. However, one thing these philosophers haven't noticed is that a knowledge argument can be constructed based on an animal subject lacking any introspective faculties, like a dog or a cat, leaving their colorless environment for the first time, except, of course, for the bit about knowledge of neuroscience, but that should be irrelevant from the point of view of the defenders of the argument since anyway they think that this knowledge does not bring about knowledge of what it is like. You can't really seriously reply saying "yes, but the dog does not have neuroscientific knowledge, that's why it does not come to have the introspective belief about what it is like, etc."

If, on the other hand, the alleged belief is considered as nonoccurrent, that is, as dispositional, then it is even more problematic, because Mary should have it even before seeing red for the first time. The reason is that this alleged dispositional belief's conditions for becoming a token occurrent belief is merely the event of experiencing red, and as long as getting out of her room and experiencing the red rose is not a logical impossibility (and it is not one!), the belief, considered as dispositional, must be taken as having always been had by Mary even before seeing red for the first time. It has the form "If Mary were to experience red, she would (occurrently) believe *this*."[17]

Consequently, I am doubtful that we can make sense of the alleged belief component of the phrase "knowing what it is like." So, in my view, the phrase 'to come to know what it is like to experience *x*' means 'to come to experience *x*', and nothing more. There is no such thing as knowledge of the process of experiencing, which is supposed to exist over and above the process itself of experiencing. Or, if it is assumed in (10) that there is such a property of knowing, which is instantiated over and above the instantiation of the process of experiencing by the nervous system, then the question is

---

[17] I'm grateful to an anonymous referee for raising an objection that lead me to write these last three paragraphs.

begged against the physicalist, because this assumption is equivalent to the idea that the nervous system instantiates something *more* than the experience when in the process of experiencing.

My proposal is similar to those of Laurence Nemirow and David Lewis,[18] though it is different in the following respect. Both Nemirow and Lewis keep talking at the level of the person Mary and argue that she acquires some kind of knowledge, knowledge *how* rather than knowledge *that*. Whereas they appeal to knowledge how, I do not think there is any knowledge acquired whatsoever, but only a new process of experiencing. Such processes are not properly described as knowledge or belief; they are raw experiential happenings, activities of the nervous system. The second difference is that whereas Nemirow thinks of the expression 'what it is like to experience x' as a syncategorematic constituent of the expression 'knowing what it is like to experience x', the latter expressing an ability, and Lewis takes 'knowing what it is like to experience x' to mean 'knowing the experience x', I take the latter as simply 'experiencing x'. Those who oppose such an analysis are quick to appeal to the propositionality of certain claims that Mary can make when confronted with red which amount to beliefs.[19] For instance: 'Mary believes that *this* is what it is like to experience red!', where 'this' refers to the quale of the experience. But it is equally plausible that no reference to any nonphysical quale is made, but rather an introspective belief occurs having the process of experiencing per se as its content: 'Mary believes that *this* is the experiencing of red!' is equally plausible, and it makes reference to the very process of experiencing, so it has the same content as: 'Mary believes that the experiencing of red is the experiencing of red'. Admittedly, this last belief content does not reflect Mary's apparent surprise, which brings us to a third point.

There is another belief component as well in the situation of Mary's nervous system, *M*, when confronted with color *red*. The second thing that is obviously true is that *M* will exhibit surprise when seeing red for the first time. A new reliably generated belief will be instantiated by *M*, indeed, with the content that *M* is acquiring new knowledge about the experience red, which is equivalent to the content that *M* did not know everything about red experiences, or that there is something more to the experience of red than *M* undergoing that experience, that is, being activated in some way.

[18] See Lewis 2004: 103, n. 12.
[19] See, e.g., Loar 1997.

But, though this belief is reliably generated—before accessing the chromatic environment, let's suppose, *M* has been observing hundreds of subjects in the same situation (i.e., having been confined to black-and-white environments), then experiencing red for the first time, all exhibiting surprise—nothing in the situation forces us to also think that the belief is true. Indeed, if premise (10) assumed that this belief is true, it would again be tantamount to begging the question against the physicalist.

Retranslating all this into the original, person-based formulation, we obtain an invalid argument:

(12) In the black-and-white environment, Mary knows everything neurophysiological about red experiences.

(13) When experiencing a red rose for the first time, Mary comes to have a new, reliably generated belief about red experiences.

(14) Therefore, there are truths about color vision that are not neurophysiological truths.

The argument is invalid, as (13) does not specify whether the new belief is true. All that follows from the two premises is that there are *beliefs* about color vision that even an omniscient scientist would not have, unless she experienced colors, not that there are such *true* beliefs.[20]

[20]I'm aware that the fan of the knowledge argument can still push the knowledge intuition by saying that, regardless of what I have argued, Mary becomes acquainted with the experience in a different way, from the inside. But this metaphorical notion of 'inside' doesn't make sense once we focus on the nervous system as the subject of experiences. There are no 'insides' and 'outsides' at this level. This is not to say that I am eliminativist about person-level cognitive concepts and argue for replacing them with subpersonal concepts. I only require, and I think there is nothing unreasonable about this, that the person-level concepts be applied to nervous systems rather than to the murky and intrinsically puzzling notion of a person.

4

Toward a
Well-Innervated
Philosophy of Mind

It might be thought that when I have been talking about 'philosophers of mind', collectively, as failing to appreciate our new folk neuroscience, in which the PNS is as important to conceptual issues as the brain (or more generally the CNS), I have neglected the newest developments in philosophy of mind and cognitive science, a group of proposals commonly referred to as *embodied and embedded* cognition (EE from now on). It is not a homogeneous group of theories, yet, all the proposals have in common a critique of cognitivism, that is, cognitive science that focuses on either abstract computational-symbolic phenomena in the brain, or on distributed, nonsymbolic, but still brain-confined patterns of nerve activation, and reduces or confines mental activity to these. The various EE proposals, starting from early 1990s (e.g., Varela, Thompson, and Rosch 1991),[1] have developed into a considerable literature by now, where the common point is to reestablish the mind-body-world connection that classical philosophy of mind and cognitive science have severed. There is not much space here to enter the details of EE, and though there is today a well-deserved sympathy for this approach, given its novelty and force, I will just point out that EE itself fails to

---

[1] Although some of the ideas emerged earlier, as pointed out by EE theorists, especially in the tradition of phenomenology established by Husserl and Merleau-Ponty, but also in the Heideggerian (or pop-Heideggerian, as the sarcastic critics sometimes refer to it) one.

meet the issues I have been discussing, namely the conceivability intuitions, head-on.

For instance, Andy Clark, in his latest book, *Supersizing the Mind* (2008), advertises Alva Noë's enactive or skill-based approach to experience (2004), based on what Noë calls 'sensorimotor knowledge' as "a powerful antidote to the venom of zombie thought experiments" (Clark 2008: 173). Yet, neither Clark nor Noë have *any* straightforward response to such thought experiments whatsoever. Instead, we find timorous references to the effect that as regards the 'phenomenal', it is, just maybe, not appropriate to equate it with the relevant naturalistic counterpart:

> All the vat scenario can directly establish is that, working together, the brain and the hyperintelligent vat conspire to support the usual panoply of cognitive and (*I am willing to venture*) phenomenal effects. (Clark 2008: 164) (emphasis added)

> A creature enjoys phenomenally conscious perceptual states when it has knowledge of the relevant patterns of dependence of neural activity on movement. But how can phenomenally unconscious states of this sort *be the basis of phenomenal consciousness*? This question remains unanswered. (Noë 2004: 228–29) (emphasis added)

The EE approach has all the elements needed to actually explain away, or at least weaken the zombie and other intuitions. For instance, the idea that it is an unsupported dogma to think of the brain as some kind of center of experience, and that experience is a global property of the whole nervous system, including the PNS, as it interacts with the world, could have been used, like in the case of the inconceivability of the zombie foot in the previous section, to show that the zombie intuition depends on some ways in which we tend to think of the subjects that instantiate experiences. Yet, those involved in the EE approach have failed to develop such arguments/thought experiments.

I will end with a few examples of problems in the philosophy of mind where changing from an exclusive focus on the brain to a closer attention to the PNS seems to bring about certain previously unexplored rejoinders.

I. 'It's Just Cables!'

Hilary Putnam's brain-in-a-vat thought experiment (1982) is one of the most discussed ones in current philosophy. Although it is mainly

used as an argument against skepticism, the scenario is also important when it comes to problems related to phenomenal consciousness. The scenario involves a brain that is artificially kept functioning
in a vat (BIV from now on) and connected to a computer that stimulates it in such a way as to create an illusion of an external world of
the kind we are experiencing: roads, mountains, lakes, forests, cars,
our friends, and what not. However, all there really is around the
brain is the vat and the computer that generates the signals. The
brain will think thoughts; will believe that she/he is experiencing a
real external world, interacting with the environment, and so on.
Some philosophers appear to implicitly *define* phenomenal experience or phenomenology (not in the sense of the eponymous school
of thought, but the way things appear to the subject of experiences)
as 'whatever is shared between you and a BIV', that is, whatever is
common to you as a subject of experience and the envatted physical
copy of your brain as a subject of experience. Thus, Terry Horgan
and John Tienson (2002), after reinforcing my earlier claim that philosophers think of the PNS as just cables and of experience as a terminus region in the brain, assume—as there is really *no* argument
going on—that phenomenology is what you share with a BIV:

> Phenomenology does not depend constitutively on factors outside the
> brain.... First, phenomenology depends *causally* on factors in the ambi-
> ent environment that figure as distal causes of one's ongoing sensory
> experience. But second, these distal environmental causes generate
> experiential effects only by generating *more immediate links in the*
> *causal chains between themselves and experience, viz., physical stim-*
> *ulations in the body's sensory receptors—in eyes, ears, tongue, surface*
> *of the body, and so forth.* And third, these states and processes causally
> generate experiential effects only by generating still *more immediate*
> *links in the causal chains between themselves and experience—viz.,*
> *afferent neural impulses, resulting from transduction at the sites of the*
> *sensory receptors on the body.* Your mental intercourse with the world
> *is mediated by sensory and motor transducers at the periphery of your*
> *central nervous system.* Your conscious experience would be phenom-
> enally just the same even if the transducer-external causes and effects
> of your brain's afferent and efferent neural activity were radically differ-
> ent from what they actually are—for instance, even if you were a Brain
> in a Vat with no body at all. (Horgan and Tienson 2002: 526–27)
> (emphasis added)

I have emphasized in the above quote the passages that indicate the
bad folk neuroscience that we have been talking about in section 2
of chapter 3; but, besides that, what is going on when it comes to

phenomenology is an implicit definition of it via the notion of a BIV. A while before, John Searle (1983) had gone even further and had implicitly defined intentionality, or mental content, via the BIV, setting it as a condition that intentionality is whatever is shared between you and a BIV. Searle also believes in the brain as the seat of the person and experience; here is a famous quote in which he states his original view about the BIV:

> Each of our beliefs must be possible for a being who is a brain in a vat because each of us is precisely a brain in a vat; the vat is a skull and the 'messages' coming in are coming in by way of impacts on the nervous system. (Searle 1983: 230)

Several authors have expressed strong disagreement with Searle, and would, a fortiori, have expressed disagreement with Horgan and Tienson about our being in fact BIVs as far as phenomenology is concerned. Besides the traditional content-externalists, I'm thinking about the philosophers associated with the embodied cognition movement, and the extended mind hypothesis (Clark and Chalmers 1998). The idea is supposed to be that if the mind is constitutively embodied and embedded or situated in the environment, then an envatted, bodiless BIV will not necessarily have to share the mental life of our embodied and embedded minds. Recently, Clark offers reason to be skeptical about this whole line of thought (Clark 2009), and Chalmers (2005) puts forward the idea that the BIV hypothesis is a metaphysical rather than skeptical one, so that in the BIV scenario the underlying computational/informational patterns going on in the computer are to be equated with 'the world'. However, I want to draw attention to something else, which hasn't been noticed in the literature on BIVs.

I agree with Chalmers (2005) that it makes sense to think that the BIV has its own world, and it is no less reality than our world is; it (that world) just has a different fundamental informational/computational level that underlies it, namely, the computational substrate created within the computer that connects to it. So the BIV is *not* envatted, if by 'envatted' one means 'disconnected from the world'. It is also *false* that it is disembodied, if by 'embodied' one means having a neuro-informationally connected peripheral system, neuromuscular joints and muscles—all these exist in the computer, but, of course, they are not materially the same as our peripheral nerves and muscles.

However, here is a novel point to be made, which reflects the concern with the PNS that I have been pushing so far. Even

Chalmers's idea of the BIV as a metaphysical hypothesis neglects the PNS, which in the BIV case would be some cables (metal wires, optic fiber, laser, magnetic fields, or what not, *but still cables* in a generic sense), connecting the BIV to its computer. The full truth about the BIV lies with the cables. For the sake of simplicity and familiarity with the subject, let us consider the case of pain as experienced by the BIV. We want to simulate with the help of the computer that the BIV has a body, and because of peripheral nerve damage, say, of A-delta fibers, she is hypersensitive to touch on the skin of the feet. Now, in order to exactly match what is going on in such a nervous system, and so to *stimulate the brain in the right way*, the computer will have to *simulate* (i.e., to represent to itself), a mechanism like the Gate Control Theory posits to be present in the *substantia gelatinosa* of the spinal cord. No stimulation without representation!

The computer will have such a gate control mechanism, which will mediate efferent and afferent impulses of the BIV, and therefore simulate the whole pattern of neural firings that is normally taking place in subjects with peripheral neuropathy. So the computer will contain the relevant structures and function of the spinal cord, as well as the relevant PNS structures, except these will be implemented by artificial circuits, not neurons. It will have to do all this; otherwise it can't stimulate in the required orderly way the experience of pain. But wait a minute! This means that the computer doesn't merely *simulate* nervous structure in order to stimulate the BIV, but rather materially realizes, implements, or emulates it. It creates whatever is needed for the pain process to actually take place, and it is part of this process. More importantly, 'the cables', the PNS, is the BIV's PNS, but also the computer's PNS. The only difference is that during the process of pain experiencing, the BIV's afferent impulses are the computer's efferent impulses, and the BIV's efferent impulses are the computer's afferent ones. This is so since the pain process involves sensorimotor control mechanisms (i.e., sensation and action are indissolubly connected). This means that each has the other both as its body and as its brain; the computer is body for BIV, and the BIV is body for the computer. Each of them is both body and brain at the same time.

For instance, suppose that the computer has to 'touch the skin on the foot of the PNS-damaged BIV'. For instance, the larger perceptual context is that the BIV has the illusion of lying on a bed, and his cat, wanting to play, pokes his foot. In order to simulate this, the computer must really implement *some kind of skin* with peripheral nerve terminations that are sensitive to touch, it must have *a kind of* damaged state of *some kind of* A-delta fibers, it must have *some kind of* C fibers, it must have a way to make the impulse travel at a slower pace (because of the nerve damage), and it must have *some kind of* a gate control mechanism in *some kind of* spinal cord, so that the BIV's cortex can receive the right nervous signals, and release its output via the action module to the motor nerves, via the cables that connect back to the computer, which motor signals the computer will now interpret as input, and the process can start from the beginning according to how the motor response is supposed to affect the relation between the computer-skin and the initial stimulus. My point is really simple: the BIV has so far been presented in the literature (for all I know) as a passive receiver of stimulation from the computer, when, in fact, they should be thought of as *interacting*. The motor signals of the BIV will require from the computer to act as well, so as to arrange and structure its stimulations to match the new situation created by the BIV's action. This is the phenomenon of *reafference*, whereby sensory signals result from the subjects own movements. For instance, suppose the BIV is lying in bed on his back and turns on his right side. This motor action will have to have the effect that a different part of the BIV's skin will be exposed to the pressure of the bed and to the wrinkles of the bed sheet. The computer will receive the motor signal from the BIV as an afferent signal, that is, ultimately as a sensory signal, based on which it will be able to create the right sensory signal for the BIV (viz., new tactile sensations, on a different region of the skin, etc.) and send this newly created sensory signal to the BIV. Sending this newly created signal is a motor action from the point of view of the BIV.[2]

So what are we to make of this elucidation? Is a BIV duplicate of yours phenomenally conscious? Is a BIV conscious? Does it have intentionality? Is it possible to create a BIV? All these questions have been answered positively or negatively, according as whether the philosophers in question are internalists about mental content and/or phenomenology or externalists. Some philosophers connected to the EE movement are more cautions and claim that

---

[2] An anonymous referee expressed disagreement with my idea that in fact the computer will have to simulate experiences in order to stimulate the BIV, because no one in the literature on the BIV thinks of the computer as simulating but merely as stimulating. However, that is precisely my point, namely, that this necessity to ultimately simulate in order to stimulate, and thus to re-create the whole PNS in the computer in some form or other, has been overlooked in the literature.

whether experiences can be simulated in a BIV is an open and empirical question. But if my reasoning above is correct, we can actually rule out that the BIV—supposed to have consciousness, perceptual and sensory states—is possible. The BIV and its connected computer are like two mirrors facing each other; there is no genuine information in the compound system. The electric nerve impulses are embedded in electric nerve impulses, which in turn are embedded in electric impulses again, not in anything like a world, or reality. This is true even if we accept Chalmers's point that the BIV is a metaphysical scenario. To see this, remember the discussion of the GCT approach to pain mechanisms. Melzack and Wall pointed out that *there is* a conceptual connection between a nerve fiber type being nociceptive and its being a pain-specialized fiber; that's how these fibers actually got their identity conditions postulated by neuroscientists. Yet, in our thought experiment with the BIV pain there is no stimulus that we can properly consider as *noxious* (or thermal, or tactile, or whatever). For that you need a world, in the sense of an *extra-neural reality*. The computer does not bring about such a reality; computer and BIV are caught in an infinite recursive reflection of meaningless electric signals.

II.   Functionalist Troubles?

Functionalism based on the idea of understanding mental states as causal roles or causal role fillers is widely and implicitly assumed in the philosophy of mind. The quotations I have provided so far all indicate the assumption that experience is something caused by stimulation and causing motor response. One could find hundreds of other quotes that indicate this assumption. The problem is not with causation or causal role as such, but with the specific place mental states are posited as occupying in a causal chain. What causes trouble for functionalism is that mental states are taken as brain states occupying a role between sensory stimulation and motor response. Ordinarily, philosophers understand functionalism as stating that mental states are states caused by stimuli and, together with other mental states, cause behavior. What is not made explicit, but is implicitly present in how philosophers understand functionalism, is the assumption or prejudice against the PNS being part of mental states; the assumption is that mental states are states of the brain caused by external stimuli *and* excitations in the afferent PNS and causing excitations in efferent PNS and behavior.

If instead we adopt a different picture, one according to which the PNS is no less part of mental states than the CNS, some troubles of functionalism can easily be avoided. According to the new picture, it is still true that mental states are states caused by stimuli and causing behavior, but 'stimulus' and 'behavior' are understood differently. Stimulus is understood as an event external to the nervous system (e.g., a burn of the skin, a gallbladder stone stuck in the mucosal fold, light hitting the surface of the eye, etc.). Behavior is understood as a bodily event occurring posterior to the neuromuscular junction, hence outside the nervous system (e.g., a contraction of the biceps muscle, a contraction of the gallbladder's *muscularis* layer, a motion of the eyeball). Mental states are then states occupying the causal role between such kinds of events. I will briefly present the solutions to four problems with old functionalism, based on this new understanding of causal role.

A. The Mad Pain Problem

David Lewis combines an analytic version (or commonsense) causal role functionalism with the identity thesis, according to which to be in pain means to be in a state with the pain-role, which by actual empirical identification will entail that to be in pain is to be in a certain brain state. Lewis (1980) recognizes that what he calls 'mad pain' is a problem for the functionalist part of the theory, assuming the pain-brain state identification is correct:

> There might be a strange man who sometimes feels pain, just as we do, but whose pain differs greatly from ours in its causes and effects. Our pain is typically caused by cuts, burns, pressure, and the like; his is caused by moderate exercise on an empty stomach. Our pain is generally distracting; his turns his mind to mathematics....In short, he feels pain but his pain does not at all occupy the typical causal role of pain....[M]y opinion that this is a possible case seems pretty firm. If I want a credible theory of mind, I need a theory that does not deny the possibility of mad pain. ([1980] 2000: 110)

Mad pain is indeed conceivable if, as Lewis presupposes, pain is a brain state merely causally connected to the PNS excitation, rather than being partly constituted by these. Lewis prefers to keep the idea of pain as a narrowly understood neural state, to mean 'brain state', and turns the initial functionalist definition of pain into a population-relativized version, according to which all we can properly define is 'pain-relative-to-a-population'. So the mad pain is just normal pain relative to the mad population, because relative to that population the mad causal role is the normal one. Lewis move is ad-hoc and the resulting theory very inelegant; no wonder it has never become popular among functionalists.

The solution to the mad pain problem is simple. Mad pain is a logical impossibility. Pain is not a brain state or even a CNS state, but a global state of the entire nervous system. The PNS activities are partly constitutive of the state of pain, hence the strange man Lewis describes is not in pain at all, because moderate exercise on an empty stomach does not induce excitation in nociceptive peripheral nerves (whatever nerves are acted on by moderate exercise, they don't deserve the name "nociceptive fibers"), and because the motor response of, say, turning one's body, gaze, and so on toward some mathematical formula written on a paper is not a pain-specific motor response (whatever motor nerves are activated, they don't deserve the name "pain-specific motor peripheral nerves").

B.   The Problem of Pseudo-Normal Vision

A classic argument against functionalism is the conceivability of color spectrum inverted pairs of people, that is people who are functionally identical, but have their phenomenal color experiences spectrum inverted; for instance, they both respond to the same color stimulus, say, red, in the same way, but one experiences red phenomenally, the other experiences green. Some functionalists might try to show that there is some deep logical incoherence at play. However, Martine Nida-Rümelin ([1996]) argued that spectrum inversion is to be taken seriously even empirically, as there are cases of inherited vision defects that seem to point to the *actuality* of inverted people.

Nida-Rümelin's case is that of pseudo-normal vision. There are three types of photoreceptors, called 'cone cells', on the retina that play a role in human color vision (in bright light conditions): R-, G-, and B-cones (from red, green, and blue).[3] They are morphologically distinguishable and normally each of them contains different photopigments, which absorb certain wavelengths of the incoming light, so that after this filtering the output nerve signal that is transmitted to the optic nerve will normally be different for different perceived colors. What colors are perceived is determined by the interaction among these three cone types. Red-green color blind

---

[3] Hence, human color perception is trichromatic (i.e., based on three basic colors: red, green, and blue). However, there are several studies that indicate there might be tetrachromat humans as well.

subjects (i.e., those who can't distinguish red and green) have their R- and G- cones containing the same photopigments. However, there are two types of such partial color blindness: (A) when the green photopigment is contained in both the G and the R cones, and (B) when the red photopigment is contained in both the G and R cones. The genes responsible for case (A) and (B) can in rare cases be present in one and the same person, thus such persons, called 'pseudo-normal', although not visually defective in terms of normal color discriminations, have their photopigments swapped between the G and R cones. Hence, according to Nida-Rümelin, they are actual cases of spectrum inversion.

But why does Nida-Rümelin think that these people are spectrum-inverted rather than just normal subjects, but whose red and green experiences are realized by different nervous system structures, a difference based on the G-cones, rather than R-cones, being involved in red experiences, and R-cones, rather than G-cones, being involved in green experiences? If what I have been arguing so far is right, then the PNS parts involved in color vision—in our case the G- and R-cones and the photopigments they contain—play a *constitutive* role in color vision. If I am right, G-cones get their name 'G-cone' in virtue of containing the green-sensitive photopigments; *mutatis mutandis* for R-cones. The point is the same as the one I made in connection with nociceptors: they deserve the name to the extent that they respond to noxious stimuli. Nida-Rümelin's idea that pseudo-normal vision is spectrum-inversion is precisely based on assuming that the PNS components are merely *causing* red or green experiences, the experience is a point *terminus* in the CNS, 'unaware of' what is happening at the level of G-cones and R-cones:

> the proposal violates the widely accepted principle of supervenience for mental properties upon the relevant physiological properties. Since the neural hardware is not affected by exchanging photopigments, we must assume that the physiological state produced by a specific pattern of stimulation of concrete photoreceptors in a given person is the same regardless of whether the photopigments are reversed. . . . [It] entails the prediction that the *very same* physiological state will lead to a red-sensation in the one case and to a green-sensation in the other. Since the only difference between the two cases lies in the way the physiological state is *caused* (by different patterns of light stimuli) and since the brain does not have any access to this information, this would seem rather mysterious. (emphasis in original)

Of course, Nida-Rümelin is right against the functionalist to the extent that both of them assume that the experience is supposed to be brain-bound, hence supervene on the brain states—that's what she means in the above quote by 'relevant physiological properties' and 'neural hardware'. *If the old functionalist agrees that when I experience green, the pseudo-normal person experiences red*, then the old functionalist is committed to the lack of supervenience of experience on what the functionalist takes as the relevant physiological state, namely, a brain state. The above 'if', however, becomes a big 'if', in the context of our approach.

My proposal is that 'relevant physiological properties' and 'neural hardware' include the PNS. To consider an example, I and a pseudo-normal person are presented with a green object. What happens is that the G-cones on my retina are activated *in virtue of containing G-photopigment*. The R-cones in the pseudonormal person are activated *in virtue of containing G-photopigment*. Both of us see the object as green. Hence, there are no pseudo-normal people: both normal and 'pseudo-normal' subjects are functionally and experientially identical.

Nida-Rümelin is actually aware of such a response, when she says that a functionalist might respond that in a normal person who *becomes* pseudo-normal

> [T]hose individual receptors that were R-cones before the inversion of photopigment distribution in the retina of the person at issue, *turned into* G-cones. (1996: 104) (emphasis in original)

She finds this 'unacceptable' (p. 103), because "color vision science predicts such a person will experience and report a radical change in his color perception" (p. 104). Now, the truth is that vision science would in such a case predict verbal reports of radical changes in color perception only if the morphological differences between R-cones and G-cones make a difference to whether they are really G-cones and R-cones, *as far as their contribution to experience is concerned*. If being a G-cone as far as experiences are concerned is essentially being a G-cone as far as morphology is concerned, then a G-cone turning into an R-cone (to the extent that it can turn into one) will result in radical differences in experience. But the truth is that morphology does not play an essential role in the nature of the G-cones or R-cones as far as their role in experiences is concerned. What *does* play the only essential role is the photopigment; so a photoreceptive cell deserves the name 'G-cone' in virtue of containing the G pigment. By far the best proofs for this claim are two facts about research in morphological differentiation of photoreceptor cones:

- The relevant types of cones had been postulated and named about 100 years before any method to morphologically differentiate them became available.[4]
- Even to this day, there are no reliable methods to morphologically distinguish the cone types without first distinguishing them in terms of the light-pigment interactions.[5]

C. The China-Brain Problem

Ned Block's famous China-brain thought experiment ([1978] 2002) is supposed to boost the intuition that functional duplication of a phenomenally conscious system does not necessarily amount to phenomenal duplication of that system. Let me first quote a passage from Block:

> Imagine a body externally like a human body, say yours, but internally quite different.... Suppose we convert the government of China to functionalism, and we convince its officials that it would enormously enhance their international prestige to realize a human mind for an hour. We provide each of the billion people in China (I chose China because it has a billion inhabitants) with a specially designed two-way radio that connects them in the appropriate way to other persons and to the artificial body mentioned in the previous example.... Surely such a system is not physically impossible. It could be functionally equivalent to you for a short time, say an hour. ([1978] 2002: 96)

Block then claims that although the China-brain system is functionally equivalent to you, one might still coherently doubt that the system is conscious in the phenomenal sense. So, phenomenal consciousness is not necessitated by functional facts.

I think that why most people got moved by this thought experiment is because they focused their attention on the wrong side of the China system, namely on the brain. Block says that the govern-

---

[4] In 1802 Thomas Young postulated the existence of three types of photoreceptors in the eye, each responsible for detecting different ranges of wavelengths in the visible spectrum. The theory of trichromatic vision was developed in 1860 by Hermann von Helmholtz, in his *Handbuch der physiologischen Optik*, and this is the time when the R-, G-, and B- cones get their name. See Cahan 1993, part I. The existence of the cones was shown later, in the 1950s.

[5] The composition of cells is frequently obtained by light-dependent histochemical staining of the optically intact, or freshly excised eye, or of isolated retina *in vitro*. Alternatively, laser interferometry on the intact eye is performed. So the availability of morphological data that differentiate the cone types depends on interactions at the level of their pigment in the first place. See, for instance, Dacey and Lee (1994) for in vitro histochemical staining, and Roorda and Williams (1999) for laser interferometry.

ment of China can realize a human mind for an hour; I agree, but they can realize the human mind only because the CNS system they create is still connected to my body, to my PNS, that is.

I propose a thought experiment within this thought experiment. Suppose the government of China is a bit less ambitious and is content with only realizing a brief pain sensation via a system of people and radio transmitters. What happens is that I offer my nociceptive nerves and the corresponding motor nerves to be used by China for the experiment. They will put me to sleep, disconnect my pain-related PNS components from my brain and connect them to the China-pain CNS system. I will wake up, suppose, with all the other cognitive components intact, except for those involved in the sensation of pain. Intuitively, I will be zombified, pain-wise: I won't feel pain; yet, when my skin is hurt, my relevant muscles will contract and I will avoid the stimulus, I will scream, and so on.

What about the CNS states in the China-pain system? If in Block's experiment you intuited that the China-brain system is not conscious, you will intuit here that the China-pain system is not in pain.

I also intuit that in this case I am not in pain and the China-pain system is not in pain either. Yet, I do not intuit that there is no pain at all instantiated by the composite system of my body (PNS) + China-pain (CNS). To boost this intuition, consider a little change to the story. My PNS components are disconnected from my brain, just as before. But they are now connected to another person's pain-related CNS components; call that person 'John'. John's pain-related PNS components are disconnected from his brain, and left unconnected to anything. Suppose there is an intense mechanical action of a nasty stone in my gallbladder. As a result, my body bends, and I scream. But, as I said earlier, intuitively I'm not in pain, since I lack the CNS component of pain. The CNS component of this process is to be found in John's brain. Now, if we reconsider Melzack and Wall's assertion to the effect that 'the thalamus, the limbic system, the hypothalamus, the brain-stem reticular formation, the parietal cortex, and the frontal cortex are all implicated in pain perception', then all these components of the pain process are now in John's brain. These structures are responsible for awareness of one's pain.

So is John feeling pain? I think the only puzzle here is whether what John is aware of as pain is *his* pain, or *my* pain, or *no one's* pain. In other words, the only puzzle that arises at this point is related to the question of *who* is in pain, not *whether* something is in pain, or whether there is pain somewhere in the global system <JOHN + ME>. *Who*-puzzles are puzzles to the extent that we take persons or mental entities seriously. But if we go back to our folk neuroscience and focus on nervous systems as subjects of pain, then my puzzle with John is less of a puzzle. We could call my nervous system S_i and John's S_j. We *do* intuit that neither S_i, nor S_j is unquestionably in pain, but only because we are not sure what to consider as part of S_i and S_j, respectively. Mereologically, the CNS component of the pain is in S_j, but in terms of neural networks it is both in S_i and in S_j. But all this indecision on how to demarcate S_i from S_j when it comes to the pain sensation can be resolved if we define a third system, S_k, as the neural network containing my pain-related PNS components, PNS_i, and John's connected CNS component, CNS_j. My intuition is that just because this system transcends the normal boundaries of nervous systems in living organisms, it doesn't mean that it does not instantiate, or *might* fail instantiate pain. It is active in the right way, so it is in pain. To say otherwise is to say that a colorful image contained in a JPG file on my hard disk becomes black-and-white just because it is transferred to an external hard disk. And to insist that, still, even if the system is in pain, it is not, or *might* not be in *phenomenal* pain is, again, to commit oneself to a funny notion of phenomenal pain as having nothing to do with ordinary pain. More importantly, to appeal to primitive phenomenality intuitions at this point, when the very question of phenomenality depends on what to say about the China-pain system in light of what we say about the John-me system, is tantamount to begging the question.

Now, the case with the China-pain system is no different from the case with John's CNS pain system. So the only puzzle about the original China-brain system is a puzzle about *who* is conscious, not about *whether* there is any consciousness somewhere in the global <MY BODY + CHINA-BRAIN> system.

D. The Triviality Problem

One of the arguments against functionalism about mental states is that it is a trivial claim, so that functional organization does not distinguish the mind from intuitively nonmental entities. The thesis is sometimes put as follows: even a bucket of water sitting in the sun is causally complex enough for there to be an interpretation of its states that would correspond to a realization of a human mind (Godfrey-Smith 2009: 273–74). To put it differently, since according to functionalism mental states are to be individuated by the their place in an abstract causal structure including inputs, outputs, and internal states, there is no reason to think that only brains could serve this purpose, but any physical system that is complex enough to be interpreted as having all the relevant possible functional states and the rules that govern their occurrence, as specified by a state transition matrix. If the world contains many such physical systems that are not intuitively minds, then functionalism does not say anything interesting about the mind, as it cannot distinguish it from any complex enough systems. Several authors have offered various such triviality arguments against functionalism. I will focus here on the most recent such argument, by Godfrey-Smith, which is supposed to improve upon earlier versions. He offers a new triviality argument based precisely on the idea that what he calls "transducer layer," that is, the far side fringes of the PNS, and actually the whole PNS as such, was not taken into consideration by earlier arguments. The argument is that any structurally and causally complex enough brainlike physical system (what Godfrey-Smith calls "control system," and what we more naturally call a CNS) could be a mind as far as functionalism is concerned, because adding a relevant PNS to it does not change some of its mental properties, given that it is plausible to think that some such mental properties are indeed PNS-independent. The crucial premise here is, of course, that there is mentality without or independent of the PNS, and denying and considering this premise a prejudice is precisely what this book is about. Here is a quote from Godfrey-Smith that exhibits this prejudice:

> A bucket of water cannot possibly have the same functional profile as a human agent, as it does not have the right input–output properties. But we now look at the possibility of taking a functionally characterized system and *changing* its transducer layer, while keeping the control system intact. This is done by changing the physical devices that interface with external objects. We might alter the hair cells in the ear so they are not moved by vibrations, but by magnetic fields. We might have muscle fibers moving a mouse on a computer screen. Altering transducer layers has important therapeutic possibilities for people with sensory and motor disabilities.
>
> When the transducer layer of an intelligent system is altered, what are the consequences for its psychological properties? ... There may be many psychological changes implied, but it is natural to think there are *some* mental features of an agent that depend only on the properties of the control system, and are unaffected by the properties of the transducer layer....

But if a system has non-marginal mental properties, a mere change to its transducer layer should not alter this fact. Two functionally similar systems that differ only in physical make-up and transducer layer must either both have, or both not have, non-marginal mental properties. So if the bucket of water lacks only the right transducer layer to be a functional duplicate of A [N.B. *a human agent*], then it must already have some non-marginal mental properties. (2009: 285–87)

Godfrey-Smith's talk about "non-marginal mental properties"—by which he means mental properties that would not be had by, say, a worm, because an alteration to its PNS would essentially alter its mind—is the perfect symptom of CNS-fixation that is so widespread in contemporary philosophy of mind. Why assume that the mind does not essentially and constitutively include the PNS, the transducer layer, to use Godfrey-Smith's terminology? Why assume that there is a difference in kind between our minds and worms'?[6] Be that as it may, once we take the PNS seriously, the solution to the triviality problem is quite simple and elegant. The "margins of the mind" (i.e., the PNS) are as much part of the mind as the so-called "central mind" (i.e., the CNS or the brain).

The reason the bucket of water is not conscious is precisely because, however complex it is internally, it lacks a PNS that would lawfully respond to stimuli, connect to the water's internal states, and be caused by the latter to set an effector in motion, say, a musclelike tissue. If we added such a PNS to the bucket, it *would* indeed be conscious. Having the right PNS-like structure is what makes a relevant complex system count as a *nervous system*. Suppose we added to the micro-structurally sufficiently complex quantity of water in the bucket a PNS-like sensory-motor anatomical structure. For that matter, let's connect two anatomically complete human arms, with intact nociceptive nerve fibers and intact motor fibers to

[6] The brain-fixation prejudice in the philosophy of mind is also, in my opinion, the ground for another widely held prejudice; the view that phenomenal states are only instantiated by higher animals. Virtually all contemporary philosophers claim, without any argument, that dogs can certainly feel pain, but "simple" organisms like worms or slugs most probably do not have phenomenal states whatsoever. Now, to think that worms and slugs are neurologically simple is another blunder of contemporary, scientifically uninformed philosophy. To take as an example the current "superstar" nematode worm—superstar, because it was the first multicellular organism to have its genome completely sequenced, by 1998, and is widely used as a model organism—the 1 mm long *Caenorhabditis elegans* exhibits a nervous system of 302 neurons and a sensorimotor system with very complex connectivity patterns. For a dynamic interactive online visualization of these connections within the worm's neural network, see http://wormweb.org/.

the bucket of water, in such a way that whenever we effect some damage to the skin of the hands, the hands will move away, in specific ways, from the source of the noxious stimulus. Does the hand feel pain? Well, it responds to painful stimuli; it has the specific specialized sensors. So, of course, it does. Does it mean that the bucket feels pain? Not exactly, but close: the <bucket + PNS> nervous system *is indeed in pain.* The whole intuition that buckets of water sitting in the sun are not minds is present only to the extent that a properly connected PNS is lacking, which makes the bucket itself not count as a nervous system. But the same is true for the brain: were it not properly connected to a PNS, it would not count as a mind. The triviality arguments work against the old functionalism, which is based on the brain-fixation prejudice, but, as I have argued, the new CNS + PNS involving functionalism is a very plausible theory and it is immune to the triviality objection.

Part II

Bounds of Mind

5

Semantic Externalism

Philosophers of mind sometimes ask questions of the sort: What are the boundaries of the mind? How far does the mind extend, as compared to the brain or the whole body? If what I said in chapter 1 is correct, the mind extends as far as the standard, healthy individual's entire nervous system, including the PNS, does. There is something to be said about the neuromuscular junction, the chemically mediated bridging between the fringes of the PNS and the muscles; as I explained in chapter 1, the parts of the body that are phenomenologically part of me are the parts that get innervated, whereas if any material close to my nervous system is merely non-neuro-functionally (e.g., by blood vessels, musculoskeletal continuity) connected to my innervated body, that material is already part of the external world. Although still phenomenologically external to me, some parts of the external world are such that I have an intimate grip on them. My case with the peripheral neuropathy in chapter 1 illustrates how even a part of one's body can become phenomenologically external to oneself. When that happens, one comes to have merely an intimate grip on that part of one's body—as one has in general an intimate grip on the world via the PNS—and that part ceases to feel as part of one's own self.

I would like to motivate and test the above view that the mind extends as far as the PNS does. In order to do this, we will have to address the issues in the debate over externalism versus internalism about mental states with content. In the first section I will discuss the classic thought experiment that is supposed to buttress the intuition of semantic externalism, the Twin Earth story by Hilary Putnam, and will articulate the three main theses of the view I advocate. In the second section I argue for my first thesis, the anti-narrowness claim, that is, the claim that meaning is not determined by narrow psychological states, understood as subjective appearances, independent of world-involving veridicality. This claim is congenial to Putnam's externalism, but only in its anti-narrowness component, and not in its positing of wide content. In the same section I also motivate my second claim, namely, that intension does determine extension. The argument is based on a definition of intension. The third section offers arguments against Putnam's wide content. In arguing for my anti-wideness claim, I consider several problems that the positing of wide content involves and conclude that externalism is marred by insuperable counterintuitive consequences; it is therefore to be rejected. In the final sections, I elaborate my own view, according to which it is the causal link between environment and the individual's nervous system that constitutes what is essential to and determiner of meaning of mental states with content. I propose a novel reevaluation of the extant issues, which will vindicate the borders of the PNS as the bounds of the mind.

I.   *Twin Earth*

Semantic externalism has its origins in Hilary Putnam's seminal paper, "Meaning and Reference" (1973). Putnam's argument is aimed at the universally shared Fregean thesis that intension or sense of a predicate determines its extension or reference. The sense of a predicate is a concept, and Putnam argues that it has a dual nature. On the one hand, it is, following Frege, an abstract object that is shareable by all competent users of the concept, and not, as it used to be understood pre-Frege, a private psychological entity. On the other hand, *grasping* a concept *is* "an individual psychological act" (p. 700). Frege, in his "On Sense and Reference" forcefully argued that sameness of reference does not ensure sameness of meaning; hence, there is more to meaning than reference. Take one of Frege's examples, the singular terms "The Evening Star" and "The Morning Star." They have the same reference, as they were discovered to name the same planet, namely Venus. Yet, learning that the Evening Star is identical to the Morning Star was, and is for those who still do not know it, highly informative, or cognitively significant. In saying that such an identity is cognitively significant we are in effect comparing it with other identity statements, which are trivial, for instance, any self-identity statement of the form $a = a$. In order to explain the difference between uninformative and informative identities, Frege introduced the notion of sense, as distinct from reference, which is at least equally important to the meaning of a term. If all identities are treated semantically as relations between what the terms refer to, we would only have trivial such statements because at the level of reference all identities are trivial self-identities. So we need a further aspect to the meaning of these terms, on top of the referential aspect, which would make informative, cognitively significant identities possible. The distinction between sense and reference will, of course, apply to general terms as well, not only to singular ones as in the above example. In the case of predicates, the reference is an extension, and the sense is an intension or concept. To exemplify, consider the predicate 'is red'. Its extension is the class of things that the predicate applies to, that is, the class of red things, like fire extinguishers, public mailboxes, and any other thing that happens to be red. Its intension or concept is the way users of the term think about the extension of 'is red', which is by way of the property of *being red*. There is a worn-out example of how a shared extension of two predicates is compatible with difference at the level of their intension, and hence a difference at the level of their meaning: 'is a creature with a heart' and 'is a creature with a kidney'. I leave it to the reader to figure out other such examples meant to show that extension does not determine intension, property, concept, and meaning.

From the examples above, we have learnt that sameness of reference does not guarantee sameness of sense, and hence sameness of meaning. But what about the converse? Frege, and everyone else before Putnam, assumed that sense *does* determine reference; in other words, sameness of sense (i.e., synonymy) does guarantee sameness of reference. Putnam's argument is to a disjunctive conclusion, such that the truth of either disjunct will equally serve an anti-Fregean purpose when it comes to the thesis that sense/intension determines reference/extension. The conclusion, which I have named AF, to stand for 'Anti-Frege', is the following:

(AF) Either (α) intension is determined by a narrow psychological state of the thinker, in which case intension fails to determine extension, and hence fails to serve as meaning, or (β) intension determines extension, hence, can serve as meaning, but it is not itself determined by a narrow psychological state of the thinker.

As it is apparent, AF is true to the extent that one has established that a narrow psychological state of the thinker is not sufficient to determine the extension of a term; this is what makes (α) and (β) stand as they do. In order to evaluate this claim, we need to get clear on how the notion of a *narrow psychological state* of the thinker is construed, and in order to see that, we need to formulate Putnam's argument for AF.

Putnam depicts a fictional scenario that will serve as a counter-example to the Fregean thesis of sense determining reference, and more exactly it will supposedly break down the following chain of determination: (a) the individual psychological act of grasping a concept determines the concept's intension, and (b) the concept's intension determines the predicate's extension. The scenario Putnam proposes is that there is somewhere in the Universe a planet, Twin Earth, an almost perfect copy of our Earth. People there speak English, just like Americans, Brits, Australians over here do. There is a copy there of everything that we have over here. Apart from a small difference, we may suppose that Twin Earth is exactly like Earth. Even you have a *Doppelganger*—a double—there, saying whatever you say, doing whatever you do here. The small difference is that the liquid they call "water" on Twin Earth is not H_2O, but a liquid whose chemical formula is very long and complicated, abbreviated as XYZ. Now consider a speaker on Earth uttering a sentence containing the term "water," call him "Oscar." Oscar has a twin on Twin Earth uttering the same sentence, call that twin "Toscar." Clearly, Putnam argues, the extension of "water" on Twin Earth is different from the extension of "water" on Earth, one being XYZ, the other being H_2O. This means that Twin Earth does not contain water whatsoever, but rather something else, indistinguishable from water by ordinary means, call it "twater." Yet, given the way the example is construed, Oscar and Toscar whenever ordinarily confronted with the liquid (i.e., when drinking it, bathing in it, etc.) are in the same narrow psychological state, since they cannot distinguish water from twater by ordinary means (i.e., without appeal to special apparatus). This means that although they are in the same narrow psychological state, they mean different things whenever they intend to talk about water by using the term "water." This further means that the individual psychological state of grasping the concept associated with "water" does not determine the extension and, therefore, the meaning of the term. To make the point even more credibly, Putnam asks us to roll the time back to about 1750, when the chemical formulas for water and twater were not yet discovered. It is still true in 1750 that (i) the extension of "water" on Earth is H_2O, that (ii) the extension of "water" on Twin Earth is XYZ, and that (iii) Oscar and Toscar, whenever thinking about water, are in the same psychological state, *narrowly construed*.

The reason I have to add and emphasize the qualification "narrow" whenever talking about Oscar's and Toscar's common psychological state is—and it is this part that makes Putnam's idea novel and radical—that Putnam's proposal to solve the above tension between psychology and semantics brings about a new notion of mental states, namely, *wide mental states*. Wide mental states are constitutively dependent on facts residing outside the individual's subjective perspective. If you accept wide mental states, then you accept that the mind is not confined to the individual—the brain, nervous system, or body in general—but it is partly constituted by facts extrinsic to it. Putnam's example is that of intentional states; states with representational content, like thoughts and beliefs. It is characteristic to such states that their content is what individuates them, that is, what constitutes criteria for their sameness or distinctness. Externalism is then the view that at least certain mental states—for instance, those that involve deploying concepts associated with natural kind terms, like "water," "iron," "tiger," and so on—are wide.

Now, by contrast, internalism is taken to mean the denial of externalism, that is, non-externalism. This means that internalism is true if, and only if, externalism is false, so internalism and externalism are taken as mutually exclusive and jointly exhaustive of the options one might take regarding the individuation of mental states. Yet, the position I want to put forward is, I take it, a middle way between the two, so I deny that externalism and internalism, *rightly understood*, are exhaustive. The view I advocate consists of three claims:

(*Anti-Narrowness*) The extension of a predicate is not determined by a narrow psychological state of the thinker, so narrow content cannot serve as meaning for that predicate.

(*Determination*) The intension of (i.e., concept associated with) a predicate determines the extension of that predicate; hence, it serves as the meaning of that predicate.[1]

(*Anti-Wideness*) The intension of (i.e., concept associated with) a predicate is not constitutively dependent on facts that are extrinsic to the individual thinker using the concept.

I will take each of these claims in turn and motivate them.

---

[1] Note that the first two claims entail the corollary that narrow psychology does not determine intension.

II.   *Anti-Narrowness and Determination*

Motivating the anti-narrowness claim will implicitly involve a reevaluation of the notion of a narrow mental state, or narrow content, and consequently a criticism of what most externalists take Putnam to have argued against.

Virtually everyone writing on the internalism–externalism debate, with a couple of exceptions, understands and asserts the externalist thesis as the view that some mental states are not individuated by facts inside the skin or the skull of the individual thinker who undergoes those states. Even though there is no mention of the skin, or even the skull in Putnam's original article, somehow philosophers started appealing to these notions as really essential to understanding what the whole externalist approach is about. This approach is wrong on ever so many counts. First and foremost, as pointed out by the two exceptions I was referring to above—Timothy Williamson (2000) and Katalin Farkas (2003)—it makes it look as though the internalist notion of narrow content that Putnam is talking about is understood as content that essentially depends on facts inside the skin or the skull of the thinker, even though Putnam himself makes it clear that it rather has to do with the subjective, first-person perspective of the thinker. When he says "meanings just ain't in the head" (Putnam 1973: 706), by "head" he does not mean skull, but first-person perspective. In other words, "in the head" is used here as a metaphor. We could countenance this lack of subtlety and the tedious literalism embodied in the hundreds of philosophy papers that discuss whether "facts inside the skin are sufficient for individuating mental states," but the problem is that it really distorts Putnam's argument and diverts attention from the real notion of narrow content, which has nothing to do whatsoever with the skin, or the skull, or other boundaries of the body. Let us exemplify with a quote from Putnam (1973: 701):

> In fact, apart from the differences we shall specify in our science-fiction examples, the reader may suppose that Twin Earth is exactly like Earth. He *may even suppose* that he has a Doppelganger—an identical copy— on Twin Earth, if he wishes, *although my stories will not depend on this.* (emphasis added)

What Putnam says is that we *may* suppose that there is a molecule-for-molecule copy of ours on Twin Earth, but that it is not essential as far as the point he wants to prove is concerned. Indeed, a few pages later (p. 704), Putnam explicitly addresses the mind-brain dualist—who anyway thinks that mental states do not supervene on anything material, so, a fortiori, they do not supervene on anything "inside the skin or the skull"—and argues that the Twin Earth thought experiment is equally relevant and damaging to that point of view. This shows clearly enough that the notion of narrow content that Putnam is focused on is not to be understood as mental content that essentially depends on facts inside the skin or the skull.

Second, let us accept for the moment that really the debate is about whether all mental states depend on facts inside the skin. This leads to absurd consequences. Suppose there is a distant planet, *Crusoe Earth*, very much like Earth except that the only vertebrate organism is a man called "Crusoe." Crusoe has a lot of knowledge about his own body; for instance, he knows a lot about his skeletal muscles—he has built various imaging machinery (e.g., PET scanners, EMG scanners, etc.) to come to "better know himself," as it were. Crusoe comes to know that the basic unit of his skeletal muscle fibers is *myofibril*, which is composed of long proteins such as *actin, myosin,* and *titin*. Suppose Crusoe thinks the thought "my biceps muscle got weaker." Now, if the skin were indeed the crucial boundary to distinguish between internal and external, then Crusoe's concept MUSCLE would always have narrow content and no wide content, given that his muscles are inside the skin, and given that there is no other muscle fiber on Crusoe Earth except his own. Never mind that we could construct a Twin Earth type of situation according to which there is a distant planet, *Twin Crusoe Earth*, that is an exact copy of Crusoe Earth, except that Crusoe's muscles do not contain *actin, myosin,* and *titin*, but three other protein types whose long formulae we could abbreviate as, say, MYZ! Obviously, Putnam's line of thought against narrow content should equally apply to Crusoe's thoughts about muscles, and prove that they depend on *external* facts, like whether the muscle fibers are built up of *actin* or MYZ. That the muscles are inside the skin does not make facts about them less external because "external" in Putnam's argument has nothing to do with whether something is inside the skin or not. Similarly, if Crusoe were to think about his own brain, the extension of the concept BRAIN in his brain thoughts would not be less externally grounded just because his brain is in his own skull. The skull, the brain, the skin—they have nothing to do with the way we are supposed to understand "internal" and "external," if we are to get Putnam's argument right. It is ever so much disappointing that philosophers keep discussing the issue in terms of skin-and-skull, as they have been doing it in the last almost forty years.

So let us go back to the question of whether Putnam's argument
is effective against narrow content in its guise as the determiner of
intension and meaning. I think that given the correctly understood
notion of narrow content, as explained above, Putnam's argument
can be made to work against the claim that such content determines meaning, although the Twin Earth example, as it stands, is
ineffective in this respect. I will first argue for the first part of the
above claim, namely, that there is a way similar to Putnam's to
show that narrow content cannot serve as meaning; then I will
argue for the second part, namely, that Putnam's original Twin
Earth thought experiment is not conclusive. The argument for this
second part will also be part of the argument for my anti-wideness
claim above.

We will change the original Twin Earth scenario a bit. Let us
think of a distant planet in our universe, call it "Stinky Earth."
Stinky Earth is almost exactly like Earth. The differences are as follows: (i) the liquid they call "water" is composed of XYZ; (ii) XYZ is
very stinky; it emits some chemicals that on Earth would make us
unable to approach it, let alone drink it or bath in it; and (iii) on
Stinky Earth people lack chemoreceptors in their nasal mucus, so
XYZ appears to them as odorless as water appears to us. It is clear,
by way of how the example is set up, that when I am drinking a glass
of water, my Doppelganger, *Twistvan*, is in the same subjective state
as I am. When drinking the stinky XYZ, Twistvan is, from the subjective point of view, drinking an odorless, colorless, transparent liquid, given that his sense of smell is missing. So we, I and Twistvan,
are in the same narrow mental state right now, when drinking a
glass of water/twater. I think this claim is not even remotely controversial. Now suppose we say "This water is so refreshing!" What I
refer to and what Twistvan refers to when using the term "water"
are distinct liquids, and not because my water is H_2O and his is
XYZ, but because they have distinct causal powers. Water (H_2O)
does not have the power to induce in me, and in all normal
Earth-dwellers, the sensation of disgust and the ensuing avoidance
behavior when confronted with it, whereas twater (XYZ) does have
such a power. The two liquids are *causally distinct*. Causal distinctness means distinctness of causal powers. Hence, the term "water"
in my mouth has a different extension than the term "water" as
uttered by Twistvan. If this is the case, then the narrow content of
"water" thoughts that I share with my Doppelganger is not sufficient to determine what these thoughts are about, hence, this narrow content cannot serve as the meaning of "water."

The second main claim of the view I advocate, the claim that intension determines extension, is based on partly defining "intension" as *extension-determiner*. There is not much controversy about this understanding. Intension is a technical term understood as an explication of the linguistic notion of synonymy: two terms are synonymous if, and only if, they have the same intension. Intension is then defined as a function from possible worlds to extensions. The intension of "water," for instance, is a function that takes as arguments possible worlds and has as values extensions of the term "water" in each of those worlds. Sameness of intension of two or more terms is sameness with respect to their picking out the relevant extensions in each possible world; hence, it ensures sameness of their meaning. If the intension is understood as the extension-determiner of a predicate, then, of course, the above argument against narrow content determining extension is also an argument against the idea that intension is, or is determined by a narrow psychological state.

As stated above, intension is defined then as a function from possible worlds to extensions, and sameness of intension of two or more predicates is sameness of their meaning because it implies that the two predicates pick out the same extension at each possible world—they are *necessarily coextensive*—which is traditionally taken as sameness of the property denoted by the predicate.[2] Now, this is all good, but it does not tell us how to find the intension of a term. I will discuss this issue at the end of my argument for the third claim of the view I advocate, the anti-wideness claim.

III. Anti-Wideness

It might look as though if we reject the thesis that a narrow psychological state determines intension and extension, we must adopt Putnam's own view, according to which it is wide mental states that

[2] This view does not always offer the right verdicts. There are cases in which we should also posit a further element, over and above intension, a *hyperintension*. These are cases when, intuitively, even though two terms have the same intension, as they are necessarily coextensive, they do not have the same meaning. An example is the pair of terms "trilateral" and "triangular." These predicates are necessarily coextensive—they pick out all and only triangles as their extension in all possible worlds—yet, intuitively, they mean different things, or pick out different properties of triangles: the former picks out the property of having three sides, while the latter picks out the property of having three angles. However, I believe that for our purposes it is sufficient to focus on cases when necessary coextensiveness is sufficient for sameness of property and of meaning.

determine extension and therefore meaning, or that meanings are not "in the head," but in the world outside, by which he means at the level of the concrete worldly constituents of what our subjective mental states are about or directed at. For instance, based on the Twin Earth argument, Putnam claims that a thought of ours having as content *water* constitutively depends on the exact composition of the liquid that we call "water," that is, the liquid that is in our vicinity. This means that our thoughts about water are always thoughts about H_2O, as that is the constituent of water. At the same time Toscar's thought when he uses the term "water" is not about water, but about something else, twater, as that is not composed of H_2O, but of XYZ. Putnam's main argument for this is the intuition that, obviously, "water" on Earth has a different extension from "water" on Twin Earth. Here is a quote from Putnam, where he asserts this supposedly obvious intuition:

> *Note that there is no problem about the extension of the term 'water':*
> *the word simply has two different meanings* (as we say); in the sense in which it is used on Twin Earth, the sense of water$_{TE}$, what we call "water" simply isn't water, while in the sense in which it is used on Earth, the sense of water$_E$, what the Twin Earthians call "water" simple isn't water. The extension of 'water' in the sense of water$_E$ is the set of all wholes consisting of H_2O molecules, or something like that; the extension of water in the sense of water$_{TE}$ is the set of all wholes con- sisting of XYZ molecules, or something like that. (emphasis added)

I would like to argue that the Twin Earth example per se is not con- clusive in showing that one must adopt the view that some mental states are wide in the sense understood above, and not merely in the sense of not being narrow, and that the argument's weak point is precisely the assumption that the extension "water" is different on Earth and Twin Earth. I am not the first to argue against this thesis; two of the earliest and very influential critical reactions to Putnam, the articles by Eddy Zemach (1976) and Hugh Mellor (1977), are based on this very idea. However, while both Zemach and Mellor offer their criticism as also a defense of the Fregean, or allegedly Fregean, perspective that Putnam argued against, my view resonates with many of Putnam's, and especially of Saul Kripke's (1972) ideas, the latter having independently proposed theses about the seman- tics of natural kind terms similar to Putnam's.

The core of the view I propose is that what is important when it comes to individuating mental states with content, and hence when it comes to determining extension, is not the external constituents of that content as such, and definitely not "any old component" of those constituents. What matters is the causally relevant such external constituents. By causally relevant constituent I mean a constituent whose causal powers do make a difference as to whether one is deploying that concept or not. Now, the concept WATER, as we *ordinarily* use it, is a concept deployed in order to refer to the relevant liquid in our environment, which we have been in causal contact with. The question is: What is it about that liquid out there that makes it count as causally relevant for our learning and using the concept WATER? Before answering this question, let us first point out that, indeed, Putnam and Kripke, as well as their followers, do relate the meaning of natural kind terms, and therefore the individuation of psychological states involving concepts associated to such terms, to a causal relation between the worldly item and the thinker. So causation is far from being alien to the Putnam-Kripke semantic framework.

Putnam (1975: 147) argues that there is an indexical element to terms like "water" or "tiger," and that the way to account for our learning the concept is via an ostensive definition, that is, by pointing to a sample of water and stating that this liquid is what we will call "water." Similarly, Kripke (1972) argues that natural kind terms are very much like proper names, and the best way to think of the meaning of the latter is by way of an initial baptism in which the referent of the name gets its name *ostensively*, and then the reference is preserved by causal interaction at every future link between speaker and hearer. Therefore, the extension of "water," as used by us, is supposed to be determined by the identity of the liquid that we have been causally interacting with. But we should notice that this last claim about how to determine the extension of "water" involves three questions that we could further ask: (i) What do we mean by "the identity of the liquid"? (ii) What do we mean by "we"? and (iii) What do we mean by "causally interacting with"? Putnam states that there is a relation; he calls it "the *same*$_L$ relation," which accounts for the identity of the liquid we are causally interacting with. Unfortunately, he does not offer an argument as to why this relation should be based on what the microphysical constitution of the liquid is. He thinks it is obvious that it is the microphysical constitution that accounts for water's individuation, but that is the very question when it comes to the issue of whether the extension of "water" is different on Earth and Twin Earth.

You might think that the microphysics-based individuation of water could be explained by appeal to the fact that we, speakers of

English on Earth, only interact with H_2O, hence, it is H_2O which should be regarded as the extension of "water." But this brings us to the second question: Who is the "we" that we refer to? As Zemach points out, Putnam has no argument for why "we" should refer only to Earth-dwellers and not to both Earth- and Twin-Earth-dwellers:

> But who are the members of this linguistic community? Whom does it include? Does it include all speakers of English? If so, it includes the Twin-Earthians who, by hypothesis, are speakers of English. Since (again, by hypothesis) water (TE) [N.B. *the liquid on Twin Earth*] is no less abundant than water, it follows that most of the stuff I and other speakers of English call "water" is neither H_2O nor XYZ but (H_2O or XYZ). Therefore the extension of 'water' as used on Earth and on Twin Earth is identical.... In fact I do not see how Putnam can exclude the Twin-Earthians from his linguistic community without also excluding Australians, South Africans, and, in the final account, everyone except Hilary Putnam himself. (Zemach 1976: 118–19)

We can dramatize Zemach's point by supposing that tomorrow it turns out that the liquid they have been calling "water" in Australia is in fact made of XYZ. Does this mean that Australians are in a different mental state than Americans when drinking or thinking about water? It looks quite counterintuitive to answer positively; it makes more sense to say that water has a disjunctive microphysical nature, H_2O or XYZ, if, for some reason, we still want to be fixated on microphysics. It does not, and should not matter that XYZ is close or far. What matters is that whatever extension of "we" we start with, it always makes sense to suppose that the liquid we call "water" is whatever we would call so based on the causal interactions we have with it. Zemach makes this point very convincingly, saying that we, Earth-dwellers, would in fact call the XYZ on Twin Earth "water":

> Let us assume that Putnam does succeed and the Twin-Earthians are somehow excluded from the linguistic community in question. Still the problem is not solved, since Earthmen, too, may call the substance in the seas, lakes, etc. of Twin Earth by the name 'water'. They will certainly do so before they become chemically sophisticated and discover that Earth water has a different molecular structure from that of Twin Earth water, and they might continue to do so even after having made this discovery. That is, they may say that what has been discovered is that some water is made out of H_2O molecules and some water is made out of XYZ molecules, but both are equally water. After all, this is exactly what we say of so many other materials: paper may have widely different chemical structures, and so may sand, and cloth, and stone,

and hair, and glue, and ... Chemical constitution is not always decisive in determining our usage of substance names. (Zemach 1976: 119)

Now, a Putnamian could answer at this point that we should suppose Twin Earth as causally and spatiotemporally disconnected from Earth, so that there is no possibility of us ever interacting with that liquid, and then the argument for wide mental states will go through. I agree with this, but then Twin Earth is pretty much like an alternative possible world, and not like an actual part of the Universe, and cases when we take Twin Earth as a counterfactual possibility are cases in which I agree that it is the actual water that counts as water.

Putnam, in his original articles,[3] runs these two versions—non-modal and modal—of Twin Earth together and thinks that the same verdict ensues as far as the semantics of "water" is concerned. But in fact they are very different. My guide here is Kripke, whose theory of rigid designation Putnam relies on. Kripke ([1972] 2006) argues that how things actually are determines what those things can be in some counterfactual situations. To take the example of water, supposing that Twin Earth is a counterfactual situation, the question is: Is that a world in which water is not H_2O, but XYZ? The answer is negative. That is a counterfactual world in which there is no water, and I agree with this answer. But the more important Krip-kean point in this context is that if *actually* what is called "water" turns out to be H_2O somewhere and XYZ in some other parts of the Universe, then water is indeed H_2O or XYZ. Here is a quote from Kripke where he discusses the case in which cats are counterfactually demons and implies that if they are *actually* demons then they do have a demonic nature:

> We could have discovered that the actual cats that we *have* are demons. Once we have discovered, however, that they are *not*, it is part of their very nature that, when we describe a counterfactual world in which there were such demons around, we must say that the demons would not be cats. It would be a world containing demons masquerading as cats. (Kripke [1972] 2006: 126)

It is implicit in Kripke's remarks that if what we call "cats" *are* actually demons, then cats are demons indeed. Presumably, then, if what we have been calling "water" in the actual world is in fact H_2O in America and XYZ in South Africa, then water is H_2O or XYZ.

---

[3] In his later work he changes his mind about the modal version. See section 5 of this chapter for discussion.

Unfortunately, Kripke does not follow where the argument leads, and two pages later he asserts:

> We identified water originally by its characteristic feel, appearance and perhaps taste, (though the taste may usually be due to the impurities). If there were a substance, *even actually*, which had a completely different atomic structure from that of water, but resembled water in these respects, would we say that some water wasn't H_2O? I think not. We would say instead that just as there is a fool's gold there could be a fool's water; a substance which, though having the properties by which we originally identified water, would not in fact be water. (Kripke [1972] 2006: 128) (emphasis added)

But this is not right in light of the previous quote. For suppose, as it is the case, that both Americans and Europeans identified water originally by its characteristic feel, or more correctly by a set of causal powers that it has on us, and then American chemists later found out that that liquid is made of H_2O, whereas European chemists found that their liquid is made of XYZ. How does now Kripke's intuition that non-H_2O quantities of the liquid are "fool's water" supposed to apply? Whose water is fool's water—Americans' or Europeans'? It is pretty clear that there is no fool's water in this scenario, but that water turned out to be <H_2O or ZYZ>.

To conclude, it is far from obvious that the term "we" in Putnam's Twin Earth scenario should refer to us Earth-dwellers. If Twin Earth is a planet in the actual world, then we have reason to think that water has a disjunctive microphysical nature, H_2O or XYZ.

However, my main point is that when it comes to the ordinary concept WATER that we deploy, we should not be very interested in the microphysical nature of water to begin with. This brings me back to our yet unanswered questions: What do we mean by causally interacting with the relevant liquid? And in virtue of what does this liquid qualify as causally relevant to our learning and using the concept WATER?

Putnam is right that narrow psychological states are not sufficient to determine extension, and I have expounded the case for this via the Stinky Earth thought experiment. Putnam and Kripke are also right that the meaning of "water" is not determined by a description, like "the clear, transparent, odorless liquid that falls as rain, quenches thirsts, etc.," *if the truth conditions of the description are interpreted as subjective, first-person appearances, regardless of their veridicality*. Yet, Putnam's and Kripke's positing that the meaning of "water" is therefore determined by the microphysical composition of the stuff is an overkill. We need not go as far as microphysical composition, but stop at the level that accounts for the causal powers of the liquid we are referring to by "water." By the very setup of the example, XYZ on Twin Earth is postulated to be a liquid with the same causal powers as the quantities of H_2O on our Earth. If we went to Twin Earth, we would call that stuff "water," as pointed out by Zemach above, and that is because the ordinary notion of water is such a causal powers based notion.

The Twin Earth scenario not only duplicates our first person *subjective* appearance of water in the mind of Toscar, but it duplicates all the *objective* causal powers that water has over here on Earth. As opposed to this, my Stinky Earth scenario only duplicates the former, but not the later, and that is enough to show that the shared subjective appearance in my and my Doppelganger's, Twist-van's mind, is not sufficient to determine what we are talking and thinking about when using the term "water"; XYZ on Stinky Earth is not causally identical to the H_2O that I have been in contact with, and hence does not account for my learning and using the concept WATER.

There is also a scientific notion of water, and that, of course, differs on Earth and Twin Earth. But, very importantly, the difference is again a difference in causal powers, that is, a difference in the experience that H_2O and ZYZ cause in the chemists on each planet. So, again, it is, at the end of the day, not a matter of microphysical composition per se, but a matter of experiences caused by each liquid in the chemists, under laboratory conditions. One of Putnam's important claims that constitute his doctrine of semantic externalism is the so-called *linguistic division of labor*, which states that nonexperts, ordinary people's use of natural kind concepts is deferential, that is, its meaning depends on what the experts have established about the extension of these concepts. Yet, this deference actually goes against Putnam's insistence that it is the microphysical essence as such that is the ultimate grounding of meaning. This is because, ultimately, the deferential use of these concepts will be based on the experiences that contributed to the experts discovering the molecules, these experiences being, unlike those of Oscar and Toscar, different on Earth and Twin Earth.[4]

---

[4] Mellor (1977: 304) observes this incoherence in Putnam's view and argues that it offers further support for the Fregean notion of meaning: "Very well. It need not be my beliefs that fix the reference or extension of terms which I can use quite well in my limited way. So I defer to experts, whose job it is to say what such a term really

Finally, let us observe that to think that the Twin Earth example works as it is supposed to leads to absurd consequences. Suppose, as Putnam and virtually all externalists that followed him did, that whenever you can build a Twin Earth type of situation regarding some concept C, you thereby show that C has wide content and that its use is dependent on what experts have discovered about the microstructure of the reference of C. To use the terminology that externalists like to use, if C is *twin-earthable*, then mental states deploying C are wide and they depend on the larger community, or sometimes on the community of experts in C. Now, it looks as though almost all concepts are twin-earthable, yet, in some cases of such concepts it is very counterintuitive to think that people who typically use them implicitly defer to experts who know more about their microstructure. Take the concept H_2O molecule. It is definitely twin-earthable. You can think of an almost perfect duplicate of Earth, the difference being that what appears as an H_2O molecule under microscope on both Earth and Twin Earth is constituted by electrons, protons, and neutrons on Earth, but something else on Twin Earth, say, *schmelectrons*, *schmotons*, and *schmeutrons*. So if Putnam were right about "water," he would have to say that when our chemists talk and think about H_2O their deployment of this concept is deferential vis-à-vis particle physicists, even though H_2O is a *chemical* concept and they are *chemists*, and that what they call "H_2O" on Twin Earth is not H_2O simply because it has a different microphysical composition, even though *chemically* it is indistinguishable from H_2O. If you think this is not so disturbing, then notice that you can repeat this twin-earthing exercise for any concept, including microphysical ones, like electron, quark, string, or whatnot. In all cases you can build a Twin Earth example supposed to show that the mental states of scientists involved in defining and using these concepts are actually never sufficient to determine "the real extension." We end up with either skepticism about anyone really knowing the meaning of any concept, or with an extreme and simply unwarranted form of reductionism according to which ultimately all our concepts are grounded in some God-knows-what hyper-micro-level facts supposed to be known by some hyper-experts. I find this simply absurd.

---

applies to. The reference or extension in any possible world of the term as we use it may nevertheless still be some Fregean function of our experts' beliefs." For reasons explained above, when I compared the Twin Earth scenario with the Stinky Earth scenario, I do not think this lends support to internalism, but only shows that it is unnecessary to adopt wide content when it comes to semantics and mental states.

IV. **Skinternalism:** *An Anti-Internalist Individualism*

The way to reject the view that narrow psychological states determine meaning is not by going to the other extreme, the one subscribed to by Putnam and the externalists, namely, that some mental
states are wide and, hence, that some parts of the mind are really
outside of the individual's organism. The right way to reject narrow-
ness is to posit the environment–organism causal link as essential
to and determiner of meaning. The view preserves Putnam's realism, which he takes as essential in differentiating his externalism
from internalist approaches, but avoids the above counterintuitive
consequences of externalism.

The meaning of "water" is a description, like "the clear, transparent, odorless liquid that falls as rain, quenches thirsts, etc.," but
whose truth-conditions are taken realistically, as objective properties out there, not in terms of subjective appearances, as what internalists appear to be committed to.

Although, on the surface, the view I propose seems to be the
same as what has been put forward under the name of *causal descriptivism*, by philosophers like David Lewis (1984), Frederick Kroon
(1987), and Frank Jackson (1998), it is essentially different. Causal
descriptivists want to save the Fregean-Russellian approach to proper
names and natural kind terms from the Kripke-Putnam type of criticism by including within the descriptions that are supposed be true
of some term, *T*, *the description* that a causal relation holds between
the denotation of *T* and the speaker who uses *T*. The problem with
this approach is that if the causal connection is merely described,
that is, it is merely the content of a description, then the
Kripke-Putnam type of attack is as forceful as before, on the condition that the collection of descriptions is taken as having subjective,
first-person appearances as its truth conditions. Let's take again the
example of "water." According to the causal descriptivist, something like the following collection of descriptions is supposed to
give the meaning of the term: "the transparent, odorless, flavorless
liquid that falls as rain, quenches thirst ... and which I have been in
causal contact with." Such a description still allows for internalist
truth conditions, in spite of the last clause—"which I have been in
causal contact with"—which means that a brain in a vat could be in
a state that verifies the description. For instance, my envatted Doppelganger, *Estvan*,[5] is in a state such that, from the first-person

---

[5] That is, a brain in a vat that duplicates all my brain states.

perspective, the above description associated with "water" holds; certainly, it appears to Estvan that he has been in causal contact with water, even though he has not.[6] The problem is that descriptivism and internalism go hand in hand, so we need a different, non-internalist approach to descriptions associated with a term.

The way to do this is to understand the descriptions as denoting objective properties, and more exactly, causal powers. What is important then is not some subjective appearance of properties, but the properties themselves. Subjective appearances of a transparent, odorless liquid are not sufficient for what, for instance, the term "water" means, as witnessed by my Doppelganger on Stinky Earth. Subjectively, the liquid that he is causally interacting with is odorless, but objectively it is stinky. How do we obtain, then, the objective intension, and hence the extension of predicates? The PNS will play an essential role because it is the receptor cells that are found at the margins of the PNS which ensure that our senses respond to stimuli properly and hence that the perceived stimuli are *objectively* the way they are represented as being by our mental states. Knowledge of properties whose instantiation is supposed to be detected by our senses will depend on our senses working within the normal range of a healthy PNS and CNS. A healthy PNS and CNS will ensure veridicality of the descriptive content of our mental states, hence, it will rule out Twistvan on Stinky World as someone whose tokening of "water" is about water. The PNS is the most important component in this equation because its margins are the points of contact between the properties or causal powers of things and our experiences of those powers. This is true even for properties that are not instantiated outside, but inside our bodies, like, pains, hunger, the position and motion of the trunk and the limbs, and so on. The link between these properties and our experience resides at the level of interoceptive and proprioceptive cells to be found at the terminations of our PNS. So the normally functioning PNS is the component of our nervous system in virtue of which all response-dependent properties, both those outside (colors, sounds, smells, etc.) and those inside (hunger, pain, kinetic properties, etc.), qualify as instantiated, so that that if there is no anomaly at the higher levels (i.e., at the level of the CNS), the experience of these properties will count as veridical.

---

[6] Of course, I am assuming here, for the sake of argument, that duplication of brain states is sufficient for duplication of phenomenal states, which otherwise is contrary to the guiding idea of this book.

The brain itself is less important in this respect. Recall that Twistvan on Stinky Earth was assumed to possess a normal functioning brain, yet, his "water"-involving thoughts were not about water, as the olfactory component of his PNS was abnormal and was creating a constant and systematic illusion of an odorless liquid. The PNS, on the other hand, is essential to the notion of veridicality. If, for instance, Twistvan on Stinky Earth had a brain which always, by mere coincidence, represented the liquid in his environment as very stinky, as we postulated it to be, his experience would still not count as veridical, and hence his "water"-involving thoughts would not be about water. The reason is that the immediate causal link between Twistvan and the liquid in that case would not work as it is supposed to, given the standards of proper functioning, which are based on how we, on Earth, causally interact with water.[7] The idea that it is us on Earth who set the standards of proper nervous functioning, and hence of veridicality, is congenial to the Kripke-Putnam approach to content, as they also insist that content is individuated according to how things actually are as far as our use of concepts is concerned. The difference, however, is that I do not conclude that mental states with content are individuated by appeal to facts outside the body. Mental states are body-bound, and so in this sense my view is *individualistic*. Yet, mental states are not internal, when internal is understood as before, namely, as having to do purely with subjective appearances. So in this sense the view is *non-internalist*. The essential point to make is that since veridical experience is dependent on the proper functioning of the whole nervous system, and since it is veridicality of experiences that determines their content, the mind extends as far as the nervous system does, namely, to the fringes of the PNS. I call, therefore, the view *Skinternalism*, to reflect the two main components of it: (a) that content is not internalist, that is, not individuated by narrow psychological states, and (b) that it is not externalist either, in the sense in which Putnamian externalism has been *misinterpreted*, that is, it does not get individuated by facts outside the thinker's skin. It rather gets individuated by what a properly functioning entire nervous

[7] If, on the other hand, Twistvan's brain were not merely coincidentally representing the liquid as stinky, but there was a causal covariance between stinkiness and the experience of stinkiness, then Twistvan's PNS would count as normal, because it would be causally isomorphic to our PNS, the difference being that Twistvan's sense of smell, when it comes to stinky water at least, is based on something other than the chemoreceptors in the nasal mucosa. As a consequence, his experience of the stinky liquid would be veridical.

system sets as standards of veridicality for our experiences involving that content.

V. Some Further Issues

There are a couple of issues that I would like to address, to end this chapter. One is the modal issue of what is the intension of "water," that is, the issue of what are the conditions for something in a coun- terfactual world to qualify as water. The other is an issue related to another popular form of externalism, namely, social externalism, or anti-individualism, proposed by Tyler Burge (1979).

As I have already mentioned before, in his earlier work Putnam ran the within-a-world and the across-worlds versions of Twin Earth together, to the same externalist conclusions. Lately, he has changed his mind about the modal version; here is a quote:

> I do not think that a criterion of substance-identity that handles Twin Earth cases will extend handily to "possible worlds." In particular, what if a hypothetical "world" obeys different laws? Perhaps one could tell a story about a world in which H_2O exists (H still consists of one electron and one proton, for example), but the laws are slightly different in such a way that what is a small difference in the equations produces a very large difference in the behavior of H_2O. Is it clear that we would call a (hypothetical) substance with quite different behaviour water in these circumstances? I now think that the question, "What is the nec- essary and sufficient condition for being water in all possible worlds?" makes no sense at all. And this means that I now reject "metaphysical necessity." (Putnam 1990: 69–70)

So Putnam seems to think, lately, that whereas the intra-world ver- sion of Twin Earth works for his externalist conclusion, the modal version is not conclusive, or rather that the questions that we can legitimately raise in the non-modal version do not make sense to be raised in the case of the modal version.

I think Putnam is wrong about the non-modal case, as I have argued so far. I also think—and this has not been addressed so far— that he is partly wrong and partly right about the modal case, and that when it comes to what he is right about, it is because of a dif- ferent reason than the one he appeals to in the above quote.

Let me start with what he is wrong about. If we accept one of the Kripke-Putnam insights, namely, that natural kind terms are rather like proper names, then we have to accept that they are rigid desig- nators, that is, that they refer in all possible worlds to what they actually refer to. It is actual reference which determines or sets the limits of possible reference. If this is so, then it does make sense to ask modal questions like "Could water have been XYZ?" or "Is a transparent, odorless, colorless, etc. liquid that does not contain H_2O transworld identical to water?" The answers to such questions will be provided, following Kripke, by our modal intuitions regarding the actual liquid that we have been interacting with. Since I accept the above insight about natural kind terms, I accept such questions as meaningful, and my answers are along Kripkean lines: water could not have been XYZ, or anything else than H_2O, on the supposition that all the watery stuff in the actual world is made of H_2O (i.e., that there is nothing like a Twin Earth in the actual world).

The part that Putnam is right about has again to do with the insight that natural kind terms are like proper names. The aspect of proper names that is relevant here is their not having a Fregean sense whatsoever, so that their meaning is just their reference. If natural kind terms are like proper names in this respect, then the very notion of intension, or concept, ceases to make sense as applied to such terms. To see this, consider that the notion of intension or concept is employed in the definition of synonymy. We say that two or more terms are synonymous if, and only if, they are cointensive. But synonymy does not make sense as applied to proper names, when the latter are understood along the Kripke-Putnam lines. It does not make sense to ask, for instance, what is the synonym of "Thomas Jefferson." It would make sense under descriptivism, in which case the synonym would be some description, like "The third president of the USA"; but I take descriptivism to have been refuted by Kripke, so proper names do not have synonyms, simply because they do not have meaning beyond reference. This means that the notion of intension does not apply to proper names whatsoever, and since natural kind terms are proper names, it does not make sense to ask in their case what their intension is, when intension is taken as the full-fledged modal notion of a function from possible worlds to extensions. I have been using the word "intension" in this chapter, and I have stated as one of my principal theses that intension determines extension. The thesis still stands, because it is true whenever *there is* an intension associated with a term, to begin with. Terms like "water," however, do not have intension in this full-fledged sense, which means that we should not worry about trying to set up and test Twin Earth type cases in non-actual worlds, as far as meaning is concerned. We can, of course, test modal intuitions about *water itself*, but the meaning of "water" and consequently the identity of water thoughts are bound to the actual world. More precisely, the meaning of "water" is its actual reference (or extension), and the relevant mental states are about water if they are about the transparent, odorless, colorless actual liquid that we have been causally interacting with. The same holds for any liquid in the actual world that is causally identical, as far as learning the concept WATER is concerned, to the Earth's quantities of H_2O, like XYZ on Twin Earth, the planet in the actual world, if there be such.[8] The mental states themselves extend as much as the PNS does, as it is the margins of the PNS that are intimately causally connected to this liquid and hence made it possible for us to learn and apply the concept WATER.

So Putnam is right that we cannot extend Twin Earth to possible worlds, but not because our modal intuitions are feeble and under-specified, but because the modal versions of Twin Earth are not relevant to the meaning of "water" and to the issue of how to individuate mental states with the content WATER.

Finally, let us address the issue of social externalism, or anti-individualism, made popular by Burge. Burge's argument is similar to Putnam's, except that whereas the latter focuses on external physical facts as what partly constitutes mental states, Burge focuses on the conventional use of terms within the larger society the speaker is embedded in. So meaning and the individuation of mental states with content are constitutively dependent on the speaker's social environment, and they are not therefore determined by a narrow psychological state of the speaker. Burge calls his view "anti-individualism," to distinguish it from the Cartesian and the behaviorist-functionalist theories of mental states, which are deemed individualistic.

Burge's most well-known thought experiment meant to push the social externalist intuition is the arthritis case. Suppose someone, John, says "I have arthritis in my thigh." Given that arthritis is an ailment of the joints and not of the thighs, if John's belief content is that he has arthritis in the thigh, then that belief is false. Now suppose a counterfactual situation in which the community uses

---

[8] Whether there is a Twin Earth in the actual world will, of course, have an effect on modal intuitions about what water could have been in counterfactual worlds. For instance, if there is an actual Twin Earth with XYZ playing the role of the relevant liquid, then the question "Could water have been XYZ in the whole universe?" receives a positive answer, because actually water is <H_2O or XYZ>. The question "Could water have been something else that <H_2O or XYZ>?" will get a negative answer, for reasons that were well expounded by Kripke.

the term "arthritis" to include rheumatoid conditions to be found both at the level of the joints and of the thighs. Burge's intuition is that now the content of the belief is not that John has arthritis in the thigh, but that he has some other ailment, *tharthritis*, and so his belief is true. But since in the two situations John is in the same narrow mental state, and it is only the conventional use of the term "arthritis" within John's larger social context that differs, it means that John's contentful mental states are determined by these external, social factors.

There has been, just like in Putnam's case, a huge literature on the subject, but I will only give a brief account of this case, based on the guiding idea of this book, namely, that the PNS is a constitutive part of mentality. The case Burge puts forward is actually pretty easy to refute once we focus on the PNS. What is the entity or fact that is constitutive part of John's belief contents when he asserts in the actual world "I have arthritis in my thigh"? What causes John to make such an assertion is a symptom that he experiences at the level of some tissues of his thigh, most likely pain. This pain has as its constitutive component, as I pointed out in chapter 3, some nerve firing at the level of the peripheral sensory nerves in the relevant tissues in John's thigh. It is obvious that since the medical community reserves the term "arthritis" to apply to inflammations of the joints, the sentence John utters is false. But it is not at all obvious why exactly it is false. Burge assumes that it is false because its content is arthritis. But this is very implausible if we take the PNS components involved in the pain that John feels as the reason why John has the belief that he expresses by that sentence. It is much more intuitive that John's belief is *de re* about the particular pain that he feels in his thigh, and not about arthritis, which is an ailment of the joints. So what John says is false not because the belief expressed is about arthritis, but because it is about the particular pain in his thigh, which John wrongly calls "arthritis." So, contrary to Burge's assumption, John's belief is not that he has arthritis in the thigh, but that he has a painful inflammation in his thigh which is called "arthritis." The fact that he calls that inflammation "arthritis" does not make his belief be about arthritis.[9]

---

[9] My approach to Burge's argument is roughly the same as Tim Crane's (1991). The difference is that Crane states that John's belief in the actual world is about tharthritis, whereas I think it is not needed and not justified to ascribe precisely tharthritis as what John's belief is about, but rather whatever ailment John happens to have in the actual world, for instance, bone cancer, if that is what he actually has in his thigh. See below.

As far as the counterfactual situation is concerned, here I tend to agree with Burge, namely, that given what the actual extension of "arthritis" is, a counterfactual situation in which people use the term "arthritis" for both ailments of the thigh and those of the joints is a situation in which they do not talk about arthritis, but something else, tharthritis. I do not have a strong intuition in favor of this view—or at least the intuition is much weaker than in the case of a counterfactual situation in which people called something else than H_2O "water," in which case I do have a clear intuition that they are not talking about water. However, nor do I have a strong intuition against it. So let us assume that Burge is right about this. As far as John's mental state is concerned, it will be about the same painful inflammation in his thigh, except that now his belief will be true, because that particular inflammation happens to fall under the concept of what people in the counterfactual situation associate with "arthritis," which is, for reasons explained just above, the concept THARTHRITIS.

The most important part, however, is that when we compare the two situations, we observe that John is not only in the same narrow states (i.e., subjective states of appearance) but in the same *skinternal states* (i.e., states of the whole CNS + PNS). Also, there is no intuition that the two situations involve different beliefs; there is just one belief having as content the particular inflammation that John has in both situations. The only difference is that in the actual world John does not possess the concept of arthritis, so he misapplies the term "arthritis" to whatever type of ailment his thigh happens to be afflicted with. To see this, consider a situation in which what John has in his thigh is a sarcoma of the bone, a cancerous tumor, which causes painful symptoms. Suppose he tells his doctor "I have arthritis in my thigh." Now, of course, the doctor will most likely correct him. But, certainly, the doctor won't just tell him "You are wrong, you can't have arthritis there, so don't worry, just go home and rest!" The doctor will say something like "Well, you are right; you do have something in your thigh, but it is much more serious than arthritis, which, by the way, does not occur in the thigh; you need immediate intervention!" What this shows is that what the doctor takes John to believe has to do not with arthritis, but with the particular symptoms that he has. In other words, the doctor rightly ascribes SARCOMA as the content of John's belief. John is still wrong because he also believes that sarcoma is called "arthritis," or that sarcoma is arthritis.

Now consider the counterfactual situation in which John is in the same nervous system state and has sarcoma in his thigh, except that in the new situation the medical community and the larger social group uses the term "arthritis" to include both rheumatoid and cancerous ailments occurring either in the joints or elsewhere. What the doctor would now tell John when John says "I have arthritis in my thigh" is most likely "You are right, you do have arthritis in your thigh, and we need to know as soon as possible whether it is cancerous or merely rheumatoid!" What this shows is that the doctor ascribes John the belief that has the content SCHMARCOMA, that is an ailment which is identical to sarcoma when it is cancerous and it is identical to arthritis when merely rheumatoid. John is now right because they call schmarcoma "arthritis" in that world. The fact remains that in both situations John is in the same mental state, with the same content: "I have a painful inflammation in my thigh and it is called 'arthritis.'"

6

Mind Extended

In this and the next two chapters, I am going to discuss some issues related to the more recent approach in the foundations of cognitive science, the group of theories that have come to be known as *embodied and embedded cognition* (EEC). I will start with a much discussed hypothesis, the extended mind hypothesis, which is supposed to show that the organism–environment boundary is largely arbitrary as a boundary for the mind as distinct from the extra-mental world, and that the mind with its cognitive states and processes could be extended beyond the bounds of the body. The discussion will occupy this chapter entirely. In the next two chapters I discuss more about what it means for a mind to be embodied and argue that most of the extant EEC approaches, though on the right track as far as foundations of cognitive science are concerned, fail to appreciate the special role of the PNS in embodiment.

There have been several papers and books to question the more or less explicit Cartesian assumption in the philosophy of mind and cognitive science that the mind is, or at least appears as, independent in a strong, ontological and epistemological sense, from both the body and the external physical environment, and maybe from anything material that is going on outside the CNS, or even just outside the brain itself. The most discussed such approach, however, has been a seminal paper by Clark and Chalmers (1998), "The Extended Mind."

There is much to welcome in this critical approach to Cartesianism and closet Cartesianism, and I will elaborate on this idea in the next two chapters. Similarly, the general approach of the extended mind hypothesis has much to recommend, and I am largely sympathetic to it. However, there are various details that I think are neglected in this debate, and whose proper discussion will lead us to a reinterpretation of the hypothesis, as well as to a new way of understanding embodiment, environment, and central processing. Unsurprisingly, the needed focus for coming to understand the issues in a new light is, again, the PNS.

Clark and Chalmers (CC from now on) address several issues in their paper, but there are three main claims regarding the boundaries of the mind that I want focus on. The first claim is that certain cognitive *processes* transcend the body–environment boundary, so these are or should be considered as extended cognitive processes. The second claim is that certain cognitive *states* can also be considered as extended in the above sense. And finally, that the phenomenal or conscious mind cannot be considered as extended in a similar fashion. This last claim is not elaborated by CC; it is rather taken as a side issue, and it appears that at the time the article was written it was only Chalmers who was more pessimistic about the phenomenal mind being extended, or extensible. Yet, as I will argue, it should not be taken as a side issue because in many ways the answer to the question of whether phenomenology is or can be extended will have an important impact on the answers to the previous two issues, the issue of process extensibility and state extensibility. CC think that the question of the phenomenal is independent from the questions of the cognitive, but I will try to show that this is not so and that, ultimately, it is the phenomenal—together with some facts about the PNS—that will guide us in what we should say about the cognitive when it comes to arguing about the bounds of the mind.

Let us look first at each of CC's two claims and the arguments meant to support them.

I. Allegedly Extended Processes

The first claim is that not all cognitive processes are "in the head," to use CC's own formulation, which they inherit from Putnam. What is the argument for this claim? CC try to pump our intuition by appeal to a comparison among three cases of human problem solving:

> (1) A person sits in front of a computer screen which displays images of various two-dimensional geometric shapes and is asked to answer questions concerning the potential fit of such shapes into depicted "sockets." To assess fit, the person must mentally rotate the shapes to align them with the sockets.

(2) A person sits in front of a similar computer screen, but this time can choose either to physically rotate the image on the screen, by pressing a rotate button, or to mentally rotate the image as before. We can also suppose, not unrealistically, that some speed advantage accrues to the physical rotation operation.

(3) Sometime in the cyberpunk future, a person sits in front of a similar computer screen. This agent, however, has the benefit of a neural implant which can perform the rotation operation as fast as the computer in the previous example. The agent must still choose which internal resource to use (the implant or the good old fashioned mental rotation), as each resource makes different demands on attention and other concurrent brain activity.

How much *cognition* is present in these cases? We suggest that all three cases are similar. Case (3) with the neural implant seems clearly to be on a par with case (1). And case (2) with the rotation button displays the same sort of computational structure as case (3), although it is distributed across agent and computer instead of internalized within the agent. If the rotation in case (3) is cognitive, by what right do we count case (2) as fundamentally different? We cannot simply point to the skin/skull boundary as justification, since the legitimacy of that boundary is precisely what is at issue. But nothing else seems different. (1998: 7–8)

The argument seems to be the following. We have three cases of a dynamic causal loop of inputs and outputs: the inputs being positions of the two-dimensional geometric shapes on the plane of the screen and the outputs being decisions as to whether the figure fits the sockets or not. It is a dynamic loop because inputs are generated by the cognizer and, depending on whether these inputs are the right ones from the perspective of completing the task, the outputs will stop the process of input generation or will allow it to continue. Since the only difference among these cases is where the loop itself is located, namely, whether it is in its entirety located in the skull/ under the skin or rather the input part is located outside, this difference itself cannot be used as evidence against the view that case (2) is a case of genuine cognition. To say that case (2) is a case of genuine cognition is to consider the input part, namely, the action of pushing the button by hand in order to rotate the figures, as a constitutive part of a cognitive process, and hence to consider it not as an action at all, but as thought. Here is a quote to show that I have not misunderstood the claim:

One can explain my choice of words in Scrabble, for example, as the outcome of an extended cognitive process involving the rearrangement of tiles on my tray. Of course, one could always try to explain my action in terms of internal processes and a long series of "inputs" and "actions," but this explanation would be needlessly complex. If an isomorphic process were going on in the head, we would feel no urge to character-ize it in this cumbersome way. In a very real sense, the re-arrangement of tiles on the tray is not part of action; it is part of *thought*. (Clark and Chalmers 1998: 11) (emphasis in original)

There is something seemingly plausible and something very implau-sible about this claim, depending on how we interpret it. It is, I gather, very implausible to say that the events that constitute the rearrangement of tiles on the Scrabble tray, which involve my mov-ing my hands and fingers, is *nothing but* part of thought, that is, as CC clearly say in the above quote "not part of action." Why I find this so implausible is that if these events are not part of action, then it is hard to see where else is there any action at all in the entire pro-cess of rearrangement. Yet, if there is action anywhere—and it seems to me obvious that there is—it is at the level of what I do with my hands and fingers.

There is, however, a less radical and, hence, more plausible interpretation of what CC claim. It is to say that while the rear-rangement of the tiles is clearly part of action, it can also be taken as part of thought. Why go eliminativist about action, rather than claiming that whereas there are clearly action-like aspects to the process of rearrangement, there are also thought-like aspects to it? The extended mind hypothesis based on this weaker claim would then be expressible as the idea that certain cognitive processes are extended in the sense that some of their components, the ones out-side the organism, though having noncognitive aspects, also have or can be attributed cognitive aspects.

Now, how plausible the weaker claim really is? The key lies in one claim that CC make in the above quote, namely, that even though we could characterize what is going on in the Scrabble case as an internal process and a series of inputs and actions, "if an iso-morphic process were going on in the head, we would feel no urge to characterize it in this cumbersome way." I think this last, condi-tional claim is right. CC think of it as a principle (which Clark in later work calls "the parity principle") expressing the essence of their view:

If, as we confront some task, a part of the world functions as a process which, *were it done in the head*, we would have no hesitation in recog-nizing as part of the cognitive process, then that part of the world *is*

(so we claim) part of the cognitive process. Cognitive processes ain't
(all) in the head! (1998: 8)

What I doubt, however, is that an isomorphic process *could* take
place in the head, "head" meaning what CC mean by it in this context, namely, the brain or the CNS understood as the *typical* seat of
central cognitive processes. Indeed, we would feel no urge to appeal
to a center-periphery type of explanation (i.e., <afferent signal →
central processing → efferent signal> type of feedback loop mechanisms), if a process isomorphic to the Scrabble tile rearrangement
were to take place in our central processing units, on the neocortex.
There are good reasons why such isomorphic processes cannot take
place in the central processing units. The main reason is that the
processes taking place within the CNS are not peripherally mediated. This is not only a piece of empirical knowledge but also a piece
of a priori knowledge: we would not call the CNS "CNS" if it were
to involve afferent signals from the sensory receptors and efferent
ones leading all the way to the skeletal muscles. The CNS and the
PNS got their names by stipulation based on what each of them is
doing: the PNS by having evolved to be sensitive to a range of stimuli ante-central-processing and to execute a range of actions
post-central-processing, and the CNS by having evolved to process
and modulate this information.

The Scrabble case clearly involves peripheral causal mediation.
It is not as if there is some unmediated causation at a distance
between how the tiles on the tray are arranged and what further
actions my brain centers decide that are needed. There is normal
PNS mediation going on, from the photoreceptor cells in my retina
to my brain, and from my brain to the muscles that move my fingers
in order to rearrange the tiles. To try to eliminate or neglect this process is to go against both hard neurological facts and phenomenologically obvious ones. This or an isomorphic process could not happen
centrally, in the brain, and not merely because the connections in
the brain are faster and more direct, as the signals travel less distance, than the ones between the PNS and the CNS, but because
such a process has a distinctive phenomenology, which central processes in the brain lack. When I mentally rotate the figures in CC's
first example, the connection between the input and the output,
that is, between the original perceptual image of the position of the
figure and the "action" of trying to rotate that image is *phenomenally immediate*. What I mean by this is that, even though actually,
as CC correctly point out, it most likely takes a longer time to

mentally rotate than to physically rotate the figure by pushing a button, there does not subjectively appear to be any mediation and time lag between the *decision* to try to mentally rotate and the *start* of the mental rotation process; the process itself is, of course, relatively time-consuming and even tedious, but the input-action nexus is phenomenologically absent. It seems automatic, direct, and unmediated.

The case is different with rotating the figures by using your fingers for pushing a button. You can actually try it out by playing the game Tetris. There is a lot more going on phenomenally. There is a clear sense in which you calculate and manage your time in pushing the rotation buttons in various ways, according to what position the figure has, which takes up time and is perceived as taking time; there is a clear feeling that your fingers hit a surface that is alien to you as the subject of experience; there is a clear sensation of a lack of full control over what the fingers do and when (you sometimes have to correct yourself after you have pushed, say, the "rotate right" instead of "rotate left" button, even if your conscious decision was to push "rotate left" button). Again, all these are missing in the mental rotation case. For instance, there is no such error as the one expressed as: "Oh, I wanted to mentally rotate the image to the left, but by mistake I mentally rotated it to the right!" Mental rotation just is a process consisting of whichever direction you actually do mentally rotate your image; there is no phenomenological gap between wanting to mentally rotate a figure *x*-ly and rotating it *x*-ly.[1]

This is why CC's case for extended cognition is not convincing. Processes that couple the brain to some events outside the brain via the use of the PNS will inherit the "alienation" that the PNS brings about when it is used to mediate between those extra-cortical events and the central brain processes. We can think of the coupled system

---

[1] An anonymous referee points out that if understood in its most general, mathematical sense, isomorphism could hold between the processes confined to the CNS and the PNS-mediated ones, just like a set of heights can be isomorphic to a set of temperatures. One such mapping would match the *taller than* and *hotter than* relations. My point is rather phenomenological and semantic. It would not be right to call a process that phenomenologically resembled a PNS-mediated one "central," even if it happened somehow in the brain and even if, mathematically, they could be isomorphic. In any case, mathematical isomorphism is, in my view, too promiscuous to serve as a criterion for whether a cognitive process could be extended; see chapter 4, section II, for the triviality problem for functionalism, where it is precisely this notion of isomorphism that makes the objection intuitively forceful.

as a whole and even as a processing system, but we can't really take it as a *central processing system*, which is what it would take to consider such a system as a case of extended cognition. The PNS is responsible for this alienation of the external, worldly processes, and the only way to argue for extended cognition would be to try to tighten the connection between extra-cortical processes and the brain in such a way as to avoid any peripheral involvement.

CC are well aware that the coupling between the brain and the external, allegedly cognitive constituents, must be very tight in order for them to be able to derive truly constitutive connection between the latter and the cognitive processing that is taking place. They write:

> More interestingly, one might argue that what keeps real cognition processes in the head is the requirement that cognitive processes be *portable*. Here, we are moved by a vision of what might be called the Naked Mind: a package of resources and operations we can always bring to bear on a cognitive task, regardless of the local environment. On this view, the trouble with coupled systems is that they are too easily *decoupled*. The true cognitive processes are those that lie at the constant core of the system; anything else is an add-on extra.
>
> There is something to this objection. The brain (or brain and body) comprises a package of basic, portable, cognitive resources that is of interest in its own right. These resources may incorporate bodily actions into cognitive processes, as when we use our fingers as working memory in a tricky calculation, but they will not encompass the more contingent aspects of our external environment, such as a pocket calculator. Still, mere contingency of coupling does not rule out cognitive status. In the distant future we may be able to plug various modules into our brain to help us out: a module for extra short-term memory when we need it, for example. When a module is plugged in, the processes involving it are just as cognitive as if they had been there all along.

They are rightly moved by the objection, yet, as I have tried to argue above, the portability requirement has a phenomenological counterpart or aspect to it, when what is needed for a process to constitute central cognitive processing is not merely physical portability, but phenomenological portability, or the subjective, conscious "invisibility" of a connection. As CC themselves point it out, their hypothesis is mostly fit for nonconscious processes, like "retrieval of memories, linguistic processes, and skill acquisition"; yet, what is distinctive about these in terms of phenomenology is precisely the lack of conscious awareness that there is anything like coupling between two distinct entities. The Tetris and the Scrabble cases are certainly not like this; those allegedly cognitive coupled systems do not involve phenomenological portability in the above sense. Similarly, portable calculators, notebooks, and so on do not pass the phenomenological test. They remain alien, thanks to the mediation that the PNS is contributing between them and the brain.

There is, however, a second part to my argument, which is related to the second paragraph in the last quote, namely, to the idea that a brain implant would qualify as constitutive of cognition, hence, why not accept that a tightly enough connected external device would similarly qualify? I actually agree with this point, but I don't think that what follows is that thereby the mind has been extended. I want to argue that if the connection between an external device and the central brain processes is made tight enough to qualify for phenomenal invisibility or portability, thereby that device ceases to be external. In other words, the only cases in which we come close to extending the mind into the external, extra-cortical reality are in fact cases in which we will have expanded the brain itself, such that even though the central processes will qualify as lying partly outside the skull as such, they won't qualify as lying outside the brain. This quasi-extended mind is in effect an extended brain, or an extended CNS.

That is, the second part of my argument considers a close relative of the above conditional claim by CC, and I do accept its antecedent. CC's original conditional was: if external processes isomorphic to the Tetris and the Scrabble cases were to take place in the brain as central processes, then we would not hesitate to interpret them as cognitive. The close relative of this claim is that

(*) If processes isomorphic to internal, central brain processes were to take place externally, then we would not hesitate to interpret those externally occurring processes as cognitive.

As I have said above, I do accept the antecedent of (*), but I also think that whenever the antecedent is true, there is an important sense in which it also becomes true that what we initially thought of as an external process ceases to be external; it gets incorporated into the internal machinery of the CNS. In their words, these cases of extending the mind are indeed cases of bringing the mind beyond the skull as such, but they also involve bringing the brain beyond the skull, so, strictly speaking, although the cognitive process transcends the skull/environment boundary, it does not transcend the brain/environment boundary; it is only that the brain or the CNS in general becomes larger and involves realities outside the skull and the skin. Of course, the anatomically defined CNS does not become bigger, but it is not the anatomical notion that is relevant here, in the discussion of whether cognition is extended, but rather the cognitive notion of a CNS. Indeed, what makes CC's thesis interesting and radical is that ordinary cases of tool use, notebook consulting, and so on might be counted as extended cognitive processes, and those cases are certainly not ones in which the functionally (not anatomically) understood brain contains those tools, the notebooks, and so on. However, if I am right in arguing that the closest we can get to extending the mind is when we actually extend the CNS, then tool use *does not* qualify as extended cognition because the relation between tool and tool user is not analogous to the relations among CNS components, hence the interesting and radical proposal of CC's is false.

Let me give a series of examples to support my claims. I will proceed from ones that are intuitively obvious to cases that are prima facie harder to accept as supporting my claim, but which become acceptable in light of the analogy with the less controversial cases.

So what we need first is a case when it is intuitively obvious to think of the brain itself as not being confined to the skull, so that some of its cognitive processes occur outside the skull. Here is the easiest case. Suppose that a proper part of my actual, anatomically understood brain is removed from my skull, while keeping all its original nerve connections intact. It can be done by attaching nerve grafts that would connect the removed part to the rest of the brain in the very same way as they were connected before. So, for instance, suppose the part we remove is one that contains cortical regions responsible for short-term memory. Short-term memory will work just as well as before, but its biological basis will be located outside my body, maybe in a pouch that I keep in my pocket all the time.[2] It is obvious that short-term memory is a constitutive part of my whole cognitive system even though its cellular support is now in

---

[2] There are two actual cases of current medical practice that are analogous to this scenario. Patients with brain tumors have to sometimes have their skull opened, in order to ease the intra-cranial pressure that the tumor is bringing about. Literally, part of their brain is located outside the skull after the operation, though not as far as in their pocket. The second case is that of patients who suffer from advanced colorectal cancer and whose natural system of waste elimination is compromised after surgical intervention. These patients, after the resection of the affected parts of the colon and rectum, are provided an artificial ostomy pouching system, by which the feces can be eliminated from the bowels into an externally attached pouch. The new artificial anus is again literally outside the skin of the patients, at an upper level of the abdomen, and functions via a stoma, an artificial orifice.

my pocket. But it is also clear that just by being in my pocket and not in my skull it does not qualify as being external.

The second case is very similar. Indeed, it is basically a version of the first. The difference is that now part of my anatomical brain is surgically disconnected from the rest, taken somewhere far, say, to a different continent, and then reconnected to the rest of the brain via a complex optic fiber remote control mechanism. Again, the fact that the reconnected part is far away from my skull does not make it less internal to my brain; my brain just got spatially scattered, but otherwise it functions as a unitary system within my CNS.

Consider now a third case. My short-term memory does not work properly because of some brain damage that I have suffered. The doctors decide to implant an artificial unit in my skull, which would be connected in the right way to the rest of my brain such as to function as my short-term memory. Obviously, my short-term memory has thereby been recovered. The implant itself is a foreign body, anatomically speaking, but neuro-computationally speaking it is just part of the brain. This case is similar to CC's case (3) in the first quote. Why the whole cognitive process involving short-term memory and other cognitive states counts as internal is not because it all happens within the skull. The skull has got nothing to do with it; it is the right connection and the right, direct, unmediated impact that the implant has on the other components in the brain that makes the implant count as *internal*.

Finally, consider the device that in the previous example was supposed to be implanted in my brain, but this time it is not used as an implant but as an "explant." The device is kept somewhere in a lab and it is connected to my brain by optic fiber, in the right way to ensure that I do have a properly functioning short-term memory. The explant stays in the same place, yet it works as my short-term memory wherever I happen to be, even when I take an interconti- nental flight. The explant counts as *internal*, for the same reasons as the implant did, even though it might be thousands of miles away from my body.

What is different between the first two and the last two cases is that in the former cases we proceed from parts of the cognitive pro- cess that are clearly internal and try to externalize them, realizing that by bringing them outside the skull we do not make them exter- nal in the relevant sense at all, whereas in the latter cases we start out with entities that are spatially and anatomically external, and realize that if they are tightly connected in the right way to the brain, they cease to be external in the relevant neuro-computational sense. What is common to all these cases is that we do have a tight connection of the right sort among all parts of the system, a connection that is not peripherally mediated, so the system can be most plausibly considered as a central processing cognitive system. If we want to put it more synthetically: whenever a case of a coupled brain-world causal looping system is close enough to qualify as a cognitive system, it is not a case of extended mind, but one of *contracted world*; what seemed to be external world becomes an internal part of a central processing unit, regardless of how far it is spatially or how dissimilar it is anatomically from the CNS.[3]

You might think the question is merely terminological, and what I have just argued for is in effect the same thesis as the extended mind hypothesis, the difference being that I call it a case of "contracted world." But this is far from true. If CC were right in their claims, then the Tetris, Scrabble, and any case involving tool use would qualify as cognition.[4] Yet, under my approach none of these cases qualify because the connection between the parts of the coupled causal looping system is not of the right sort to qualify as a *central* process, mainly because it is peripherally mediated both neurologically and phenomenologically. Furthermore, cases that *would* qualify as cognition, because of the lack of peripheral mediation and the satisfaction of certain other conditions (like portability, availability, automaticity of endorsement, and systematicity), are dissimilar from CC's main cases of what they call "extended mind" and are much less radical than their hypothesis. These are cases of implants and explants, that is, devices that interact in a peripherally unmediated, direct way with other parts of the cognitive brain system.

---

[3] Thus I disagree with Fred Adams and Ken Aizawa when they say (2008: 78): "Perhaps one day it will be possible to replace the rods and cones in the human retina with synthetic rods and cones. These synthetic cells, these micro-tools, might have the size and shape of naturally occurring human rods and cones. They might have the same neurotransmitter handling properties. They might have the same response properties to light. In such a future, there might well be individuals whose cognitive processes extend beyond their organismal boundaries, giving them trans-organismal cognition." Such micro-tools, if I am right, would not make the mind extended in any sense, even less so than my explants. Artificial rods and cones in the retina would simply be bona fide parts of the nervous system, hence, would not make the mind extended in any sense.

[4] The case of ordinary tool use, given some other conditions (availability, portability, automaticity, systematicity), is rightly pointed out by Adams and Aizawa (2008: 78–79) as the typical case of supposedly extended cognition and the main source of controversy when it comes to the issue of how radical the thesis is supposed to be. See also Daniel Dennett (2000) and Adams and Aizawa (2001).

As mentioned when I introduced CC's paper, there are three main claims in it: that cognitive processes are extended, that cognitive states are extended, and that phenomenal consciousness is probably not extended. I have so far discussed the first of these claims, so I will move now to discussing the second one.

II. *Allegedly Extended States*

The second claim is that not only cognitive processing sometimes takes place by transcending the brain–world boundary, but mental states as well. Such mental states include beliefs, desires, and emotions. CC focus on making a case for belief as extended. Here is their thought experiment:

> First, consider a normal case of belief embedded in memory. Inga hears from a friend that there is an exhibition at the Museum of Modern Art, and decides to go see it. She thinks for a moment and recalls that the museum is on 53rd Street, so she walks to 53rd Street and goes into the museum. It seems clear that Inga believes that the museum is on 53rd Street, and that she believed this even before she consulted her memory. It was not previously an *occurrent* belief, but then neither are most of our beliefs. The belief was sitting somewhere in memory, waiting to be accessed.
>
> Now consider Otto. Otto suffers from Alzheimer's disease, and like many Alzheimer's patients, he relies on information in the environment to help structure his life. Otto carries a notebook around with him everywhere he goes. When he learns new information, he writes it down. When he needs some old information, he looks it up. For Otto, his notebook plays the role usually played by a biological memory. Today, Otto hears about the exhibition at the Museum of Modern Art, and decides to go see it. He consults the notebook, which says that the museum is on 53rd Street, so he walks to 53rd Street and goes into the museum.

CC argue that the cases of Inga and Otto are entirely analogous; hence, we should attribute a standing belief to Otto, a belief that resides outside his brain, in the notebook. A similar case can then be made for desires or other types of mental states.

I agree that there is *information* in Otto's notebook; no one would deny this much, I think. Similar repositories of information are hard disks, USB memory sticks, CDs, and so on. The question is whether the fact that there is information in the notebook is identical to the supposed fact that that information constitutes Otto's belief. CC's argument for ascribing Otto the standing belief that the museum is on 53rd Street is based on the same reasoning as the previous argument for extended processing. It is the constant and systematic availability of the notebook, as well as Otto's immediate and unconditioned endorsement of whatever the notebook tells him that makes the notebook contain information that counts as Otto's own belief. In other words, it is again the trans-cranial characteristics of the *processing* that makes Otto count as an agent with extended belief states. If this were not so, then any information on any hard disk in the world would count as my extended beliefs. It is the special *access* to the notebook that makes it—the argument goes—look like a bona fide belief of Otto's.

CC's main point here is that *standing* beliefs are extended, even though occurrent ones are supposedly in the head. Clark has recently (2010) made this point explicit. I will argue that the sense in which Otto's standing beliefs are not in his nervous system is a sense in which occurrent beliefs and desires can also sometimes be outside the nervous system, and that that sense does not make it really the case that those alleged beliefs and desires count as genuine ones; and, following my strategy in the case of allegedly extended processing, I will also argue that whenever such cases do count as involving genuine beliefs and desires, the seemingly external devices involved cease to count as external.

Let me start with a real story. I'm not big on technology and gadgets. I have only got an old cell phone and use it sparingly, for talking. My wife, Ezgi, however, is much better informed and skilled technologically. She has a smart phone, which she uses for various purposes, far beyond talking, some of which uses I never bothered to fully understand, to my shame. A couple of days ago she reported, visibly upset, that she had just remembered that two weeks before she had had an appointment with a friend at *Cafe In*, a cafeteria on our campus at Bilkent University, which she had completely forgotten about. She was supposed to borrow a book from the friend, which was important for her upcoming research. "It never happened to me before that I completely forget about an appointment," she said, and then she added something that puzzled me: "But, you know, this is not going to happen again!"

I was puzzled for the moment. Did she mean she's going to start some memory- improvement exercises? But even so, how could she be sure that "this is not going to happen again"? Then my puzzlement went away, as she immediately added the explanation: "I'm going to set up a nice alert system on my phone, so each time I need to do something, I'll be informed at the right time." She has now, I think, a double alert system. One is that every morning, when she touches the screen of the phone for the first time that day, the phone tells her what the duties, events, deadlines, and so on of the day are. The second one is an alarm ring that tells her—for appointments and meeting dates that she has in advance introduced in the phone's calendar—that they are going to happen soon, say, in a couple of hours.

What I find interesting about this is that not only the alleged standing beliefs are stored by the phone, but the phone, especially via the second component of the alert system, seems to store Ezgi's *occurrent* desires too. "My friend is supposed to be at *Cafe In* at 2 pm today and I wish *now* to meet my friend today at 2 pm at *Cafe In*"—this is what the phone seemingly reminds her, at the right time for the tokening of "now." The message on her phone, therefore, contains both a belief and an occurrent desire, if indeed CC are right that these are cases of extended such states.

I am again skeptical that these count as beliefs and desires, or at least I'm skeptical that they count as *Ezgi's* beliefs and desires, though they definitely count as information. And if the notions of belief and desire imply that a belief or a desire is always *someone's*, then they won't count as beliefs and desires. The reason I think the information expressed in the quoted sentence in the previous paragraph does not count as Ezgi's standing belief is, again, that there is peripheral mediation between the information in the phone and Ezgi's CNS states. The process of retrieving the information from the memory of the phone is not done in a way that is direct enough, so as to bypass any peripheral pathways, as it normally happens when we retrieve information from our normal, internal memory. The issue is not that she does not automatically endorse what the phone says, or that she might stop and wonder whether what the phone says is true. She might well just always automatically endorse whatever the phone says, and it also happens many times that we doubt our own memory. The issue is rather that, again, the phenomenology in the two cases, the case of internal retrieval of a standing belief or occurrence of a desire *versus* the case of retrieval of information by looking on the phone screen, is very different. One involves a phenomenological immediacy, whereas the latter involves phenomenologically peripheral mediation. You might think phenomenology should not be relevant to such processes, especially because CC themselves are explicitly noncommittal with respect to whether phenomenology is extended or can be extended. Yet, it is relevant when we think about the condition of portability, which

CC consider to be important in order to have a good case for mental extension.

CC admit that the external component of the coupled brain-world system has to be portable, in the sense that it has to be available whenever the agent needs it. Yet, I think even when this portability requirement is satisfied we still do not have a genuine cognitive system with genuine beliefs and desires because it is not indifferent to whom it is available. The words of American satirist Ambrose Bierce, from his delightfully humorous sarcastic lexicon, *The Devil's Dictionary*, are spot on here. He defines the word "portable" as follows:

> "PORTABLE, adj. Exposed to a mutable ownership through vicissitudes of possession."

The gist of Bierce's piece of bitter sarcasm here is that for something to be portable essentially means that one can steal it or appropriate it more generally. In other words, ownership of a portable thing is never guaranteed. The same is true of both the alleged beliefs and the alleged desires that Ezgi supposedly possess by carrying her phone around and checking it. What I am saying might seem silly, but the phone can be stolen, and together with it all the information; and yet, it is hard to make sense of a standing belief being stolen from me by someone, so that it becomes the thief's possession.[5] Suppose someone, Jack, steals Ezgi's phone and Otto's notebook, and is going to use those external devices just the way their original possessors used to. If CC were right that the phone and the notebook served as constitutive support for the standing beliefs of Ezgi and Otto, respectively, then not only Ezgi and Otto would come to be *dispossessed* of those beliefs, but Jack would come *possess* them. While being dispossessed of one's standing belief might make sense, for instance, by erasing one's memory, and coming to *have* a new belief is also unproblematic, I am skeptical that coming to *possess someone else's*, or what used to be someone else's standing belief really makes sense.[6]

---

[5] An anonymous referee expressed the concern that although my arguments that follow below holds for the case of stealing the phone, they might not hold for the case of accidental swap of the phones. Nothing depends here on whether it is stolen or accidentally taken by someone else; all that matters is that someone gets dispossessed of some standing beliefs and thereby someone else comes to possess these beliefs, which, I argue, does not make much sense.

[6] Thus my objection here is different from the one by Martin Davies that Clark (2010: 57) quite comfortably replies to: "But why suppose that uniqueness of access is anything more than a contingent fact about standard biological recall? If, in the

What is wrong with Jack stealing the phone and the notebook *and* using them the way Ezgi and Otto, respectively, used to is ultimately grounded in Ezgi's and Otto's internal, brain-bound cognitive system: it is because of the internal occurrent beliefs that they had when introducing the information in the phone and the notebook, respectively, which makes it the case that if Jack uses the phone and notebook their way, he does not thereby come to possess their beliefs and desires, but rather, at most comes to *falsely* believe that he has a certain belief or a desire. This also explains why it is unlikely that Jack would actually use these devices the way their original possessors did. Jack would most probably not endorse "I wish now to meet my friend X...," but rather interpret it the right way, as "The original possessor of the phone *would* wish now to meet her friend X."[7] This is again because the connection between what the phone displays and what the current possessor does based on that is a peripherally mediated one, in this case by visual perception. On the other hand, a piece of information from the notebook, like that the museum is on the 53rd Street, while generating a true belief in Jack's cognitive system, is more plausibly to be taken for what it is: information in the world, on a par with so many more pieces of information that we would not take as part of anyone's cognitive system.

CC do consider the problem of portability, but only in light of the possibility of too easy decoupling. The more interesting, and, if I have been right in what I argued above, damaging problem is that of *recoupling*. The problem of recoupling is that coupled systems of the kind CC take as extended mental states are too easily recoupled and in the wrong way; witness Jack's case with Ezgi's and Otto's devices. What explains why some, and I would say *most*, ways of recoupling are wrong is, ultimately, that what did the original coupling was itself a distinct, unitary, nervous-system-bound cognitive system, different from the new cognitive system that the device gets recoupled with. If this is the case, then the original cognitive system has never had the external device as its constitutive part.

---

future, science devised a way for you to occasionally tap into my stored memories, would that make them any less mine, or part of my cognitive apparatus?" My case is not one of mere tapping into someone else's memory, but coming to exclusively possess it, while dispossessing the other.

[7] What if Jack himself is an Alzheimer sufferer? Would that make him genuinely having the desires and beliefs of Otto and Ezgi when using their devices? I don't think so. He would only have the second-order belief that he does have those beliefs and desires, and I intuit that there is nothing to force us to think that this second-order belief is true.

Finally, let me offer the second part of my argument, which is, just like in the previous section, that if indeed some seemingly external entity functions so as to be considered part of a cognitive state, like belief or desire, then the seemingly external device is not external in the relevant, neuro-computational sense. That is, it is more plausibly to be taken as part of the nervous system, and hence the case is not one of extended mind, but what I have dubbed "contracted world," a case in which a previously autonomous part of the world gets "captured" by a nervous system and so ceases to count as an external from then on.

The argument for this claim is the same as my argument in the previous section, where we discussed the case of cognitive processes. Once we ensure that, for instance, Otto's notebook and Ezgi's phone are tight enough for the information that is to be found in them to count not merely as information out there, but constitutive part of beliefs and desires that Otto and Ezgi have, it is more intuitive to consider that thereby the notebook and the phone have become parts of the brain, neuro-computationally speaking, so that they have ceased to count as external to the brain or the nervous system in general. Such a tightening of the coupling is not, I suppose, technologically impossible. What we have to do is to transform the notebook and the phone into what I earlier referred to as explants, that is, physically and anatomically external devices, but whose interaction with the nervous system is not peripherally mediated, so they get directly integrated as central processes. For instance, we digitize Otto's notebook, by transferring the information that it contains to a smart USB drive. Then we connect the USB drive by optic fiber to Otto's brain in such a way that he would never become aware, while retrieving the information from the USB drive, that the USB even exists, let alone that there is a connection between it and the nervous system. Retrieval of information would thereby truly emulate what normally happens within the brain. The USB drive would still be carried in the pocket, but Otto would never have to look at it or visually, auditorily, etc. attend to anything, like he used to do with the notebook (as a matter of fact, in wouldn't make much sense to look at and visually contemplate a USB drive, would it?). Now, even if carried in his pocket, the USB drive is a bona fide functional part of Otto's brain. It is not that his mind extended so as to outrun his brain—though spatially and anatomically it did, but those senses of "outrunning" are not relevant—but rather something that used to be an autonomous external entity has become an integrated part of the neuro-functionally understood brain. That this is incompatible with what CC claim is shown by the fact that the original Otto case, when he had to open the notebook and look at it, does not count under my approach as a case when the notebook has anything to do with central cognition. Similar thoughts apply, of course, to Ezgi's phone. It can be turned from a mere phone into an explant, so that when Ezgi wants to remember something she does not ever have to touch the screen, let alone look at it or hear its alarm. If the phone becomes such an explant, then the phone counts as part of her cognitive system and the information as constitutive of her beliefs and desires. At the same time, of course, the phone will have become an internal functional part of her brain, so we have no case of extended cognition in the original and radical sense that CC have argued for.

What about the case of Jack stealing such an explant? I think the explant, unlike the original notebook and phone, is not portable in the Ambrose Bierce sense of "portable." First of all, in the case when Jack stole the notebook and the smart phone we noted that the peripheral mediation, both neural and phenomenological, makes it likely that Jack would not use these devices the way the original owners used to. Jack would not endorse "I need now to meet my friend" and "My friend is at the cafe." Rather the right prediction is that he would endorse something like "Whoever owned the phone before needs now to see her friend" and "The friend of whoever owned the phone before is at the cafe." Not so when Jack steals the explant, which is now connected directly to his brain, without peripheral and receptor mediation (i.e., vision, hearing, etc.). Now Jack will, by default, endorse these statements, as they will be felt as his own thoughts. Ezgi's alarm ring will, as it were, ring in Jack's head now. Second, the relevant process of recoupling, after Jack steals the phone or the USB explant, is one by which Jack connects these to his brain in such a way as to preserve the coherence of the overall belief and desire systems, one which takes into account that memory is not a simple access to stored data, but highly interactive and reconstructive.[8] If this is the case, then Jack's recoupling of the USB or the phone will involve preservation of whatever is relevant from the USB's or the phone's interactions with the brains of the previous owners. Now, this type of recoupling so much more difficult and different from the simple recoupling in the case of Jack's stealing the original phone and notebook that it clearly makes the two cases count as different in kind. The explants are parts of the

---

[8] These properties of actual memory are happily endorsed by Clark (2010): "Certainly, biological memory is an active process. And retrieval is to a large extent reconstructive rather than literal: what we recall is influenced by our current mood, our current goals, and by information stored after the time of the original experience."

mind, but on pain of ceasing to count as external in the same sense in which Otto's notebook does. Otto's notebook, on the other hand, does count as external in the relevant sense, as its interaction with Otto's nervous system is peripherally mediated, but on pain of not counting as constitutive part of a cognitive system.

So is the mind extended, ultimately? Based on the type of examples I have considered from Chalmers and Clark, it is not. All the cases of central cognitive processing were, as I argued, brain-bound in those cases, and whenever it looked as though some cognitive processes are both central and not brain-bound, I argued that they are rather cases of the brain getting bigger, or part of the world getting contracted.[9]

There is, however, one type of case which I do take to be a case of cognitive system that extends beyond the brain. That is the case of the PNS, or the peripheral mind, playing a cognitive role rather than only its normal sensory role. If I am right, the cognitive mind is extended, but not beyond the bounds of the PNS. The paradigmatic case I have in mind is one that Clark and Chalmers consider in their paper as the most justifiable case of external involvement in computation, namely, the case of counting on one's fingers, or more generally of using one's finger motions as an aid in all sorts of computation. I find this case extremely interesting and worth discussing. Also, I agree that the fingers used this way constitute a good case for cognition that extends beyond the CNS, but it is at the same time not a case as radical as the other alleged cases of extended cognition. It is an instance of the more general case for the embodied mind, which is the topic I will address in the next two chapters.

---

[9] My colleague, Kirk Michaelian, has objected that all my arguments offered in this chapter are directed to the Parity Principle; however, a second wave of the extended mind thesis is based on the Complementarity Principle rather than on Parity. This latter principle does not require an external device to replicate whatever an internal, central cognitive process would do, but rather it allows such external devices to complement the internal ones, that is, the internal and the external processes perform different functions, but they count as integrated into a unitary cognitive system (Clark 2010; Menary 2010; Sutton 2010). I have two replies to this challenge. One is that, in my opinion, none of the authors who discuss complementarity has offered a precise enough explanation of the criteria by which to judge whether some external processes that causally interact with the cognizer count as complementary to and integrated with internal processes. Parity is at least a precise principle, but Complementarity needs a lot more clarification. The second reply is that my arguments equally apply to a complementarity based approach to the extended mind because even in cases of complementarity there is peripheral mediation between the external devices and the internal cognitive processes, as far as phenomenology is concerned.

Part III

Mind Embodied

7

Embodiment and the Peripheral Mind

A good discussion of perception related to bodily states and changes should intuitively be a tour de force of an essay dedicated to an embodied view of the mind. I hope this chapter will live up to this expectation, and hence I intend not only to discuss various problems related to how the body, and more exactly the PNS, plays a role in mental states, but to also put forward a novel empirical argument for the thesis that the PNS is constitutive of experience. In chapter 2, I might have given the impression of skepticism that such an argument exists, that we should aim low, and only accept that at least it is not nonsense to think about PNS processes as partly constituting conscious experience. I want now to offer a more vigorous tackling of this issue and actually convince you that there are cases when the issue of whether some PNS process is a constitutive or merely a causal element does not even arise because the only option is that it is constitutive of experience. I will start with a discussion of proprioception in general, and from some cases of proprioceptive illusions I will build my empirically based argument for the embodied mind, in the form of my PMH. To my knowledge this will be the first time that such an argument is formulated, that is, an argument that is not based merely on a reconceptualization of some notion, like "mind," "cognition," and so on, but on empirical facts that point beyond any merely causal contribution of the areas outside the CNS. In the second section, I will discuss the notion of embodiment and advance the thesis that it is conceptually linked to innervation. Third, I will discuss the alleged possibility of disembodiment, so dear to philosophers, and argue that it is not justified and that the alleged possibility, when thought through, collapses. This will vindicate my view that the mind is essentially embodied.

I. 'Fingers Crossed for the Embodied Mind!'

Let me begin with a quote that I find odd, especially that it comes from one of the handful of philosophers of mind who, unlike most others who have been vision-fixated, has extensively thought and written about bodily or proprioceptive phenomena, Brian O'Shaughnessy:

> [I]n every instance of tactile perception a proprioceptive awareness of one's body *stands between one* and awareness of the tactile object: it is only through being aware of one's body that one becomes aware of the objects given to touch. And so the sense of touch must depend upon proprioception, and not vice versa. Therefore whether or not proprioception is *absolutely* immediate, it must be immediate in ways not open to touch. (2000: 629) (emphasis in original)

What I find odd is how O'Shaughnessy follows other philosophers' way of speaking about the self as a receiving subject of what one is proprioceptively aware of. This I find weird because, subjectively, it just does not feel like this. What I am proprioceptively aware of is not my body *qua* something loosely "mine," like my wallet is, but *simply myself*. As I pointed out in chapter 1, we clearly seem to inhabit our neurally healthy bodily peripheries as much as our alleged "center," and in fact this alleged center can easily cease to be a center, for instance, when we are badly hurt in some distal part of the body; in that case the intense pain we feel is definitely not something mental in the sense of "mental" used when we tend to think of the mind as being seated in the cranium. O'Shaughnessy points out correctly that awareness of the object of touch is less direct as compared to awareness of one's body, but it is not, as he thinks, because the awareness of one's body gets situated "*between one* and the awareness of the tactile object." It is because awareness of one's body is just self-awareness, whereas awareness of the touched object is awareness of something external to the self. Finally, he is right in a sense that the tactile must depend on the proprioceptive and not vice versa, namely, in the sense that being aware merely *that one is touching something* implies being aware of one's body, or simply being self-aware. But there is a more fine-grained sense of proprioception and I doubt that in that sense it is always logically prior to touch. This second sense is associated not with one being aware merely that one is touching something, but with a more or less precise awareness of the details of the touched object. For instance, in the first, general sense, I am in the same proprioceptive state when I touch a soft ball as when I touch a hard wall: I am aware of myself through touching. I say that I am aware of myself *through* touching, not aware of myself-as-touching, which is more like an introspective state (see section II below). But in the second sense I am in different states, proprioceptively aware in a very different way when I touch the soft ball than when I touch the hard wall.

To use the Husserlian distinction between *noesis* and *noema* (Husserl [1913] 1962), augmented with Gallagher's (2005) notion of the *prenoetic*, we can distinguish three components *in* the experience of touching an object, and two components at the margins, so to say, of this experience. In the experience we have pre-reflective awareness of oneself (being aware of myself *through* touching), the noetic (the perceiving), and the noematic (the *what* of my awareness when I am touching). At the margins we have, first, what Gallagher calls "the prenoetic," that is, embodied factors that shape or color my experience, but without entering awareness,[1] and, second, what I referred to as awareness of myself-as-touching, which is a reflective process likely to require a secondary focus, based on voluntary effort.

In order to prove my claim that proprioception in the fine-grained or noematic sense is not always prior to touch, but sometimes *determined* by it, we need to consider some exotic ways to touch or be touched; namely, some cases of touching that generate tactile-proprioceptive illusions. It is in effect surprising that in his lengthy discussion of touch and proprioception O'Shaughnessy does not consider any case of tactile, proprioceptive, or tactile-proprioceptive illusions. Anyway, in what follows such cases will play an important role in trying to correctly conceptualize proprioception, and some of them will be essential empirical bases for my argument for the embodied mind, in the form of PMH.

---

[1] Gallagher (2003) offers a critical view of O'Shaughnessy's and Bermudez's (1998) analyses of proprioception, similar to my points here, and distinguishes proprioceptive *information* from proprioceptive *awareness*, where, he argues, the former should be taken as prenoetic while the later as non-perceptual, so that proprioception in its most typical, pre-reflective or non-thetic guise (Merleau-Ponty [1945] 2002; Sartre [1956] 2011) is not a form of perception. However, Gallagher notes, in personal correspondence, that there are some ambiguities when it comes to definitely classifying processes as prenoetic or pre-reflective noetic, but these are ambiguities in the processes themselves, not simply in the theoretical or phenomenological account of the processes.

Aristotle is believed to be the first to mention in writing the tactile-proprioceptive illusion that now bears his name, *Aristotle's illusion*. Thus in *Metaphysics*, Book *Gamma*, part 6, he points out that "touch says there are two objects when we cross our fingers, while sight says there is one." In order to see what exactly happens, cross your index and middle fingers (for some people it works better by crossing the middle and the ring finger), say, on the left hand (most people can do it easier with the middle finger above the index finger, as the latter is shorter), then touch the body of a cylindrical pencil to the skin on the angle that is formed by the crossed fingers, that is, touch the two fingers simultaneously by applying the pencil between the fingertips that are now crossed, as in the photo (figure 7.1).

What happens is that most people, though not all, feel as if they were touched by two objects, not one. It is a tactile version of what happens in double vision, namely, the resulting visual experience of double image when the eyes are crossed by focusing on a close object. The illusion is, of course, partly tactile, but it is also taken as partly proprioceptive, namely, when touched we fail to correctly proprioceive our fingers as crossed, and, as it is usually put, at the moment the touch occurs, the brain is fooled into thinking that the fingers

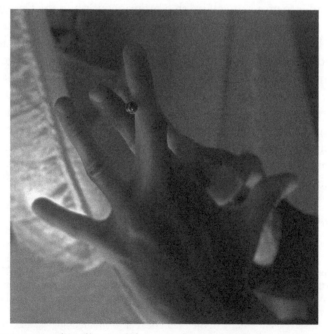

Figure 7.1 Aristotle's illusion (Photo credit: Alex Robciuc)

are not crossed, because it interprets the touch as if the fingers were uncrossed (Benedetti 1985, 1986). If this is right, then O'Shaughnessy's claim that touch is logically posterior to proprioception is false, in the sense of fine-grained proprioception. This is so because before the occurrence of the touch we proprioceive our fingers as crossed, whereas the immediate effect of the touch is for us to fail to proprioceive the fingers as crossed, so it is the tactile stimulus that determines which proprioceptive state we are in.[2] One might insist, in defense of O'Shaughnessy, that what the case shows is merely that touch sometimes has causal priority, not that proprioception is not logically prior, because both before and after being touched we do proprioceive our fingers per se, that is, as just "being there." It is true that we do have proprioceptive awareness of our fingers just being there, both before and after, but my point is about the particular way we are aware of our fingers (i.e., crossed before and uncrossed after the touch). Still, one might insist that I haven't shown that at the moment of touch the proprioceptive awareness as of uncrossed fingers is not a precondition for the touch to be felt as if caused by two objects. I don't think that it is a precondition at all, although one might take it as a *causal* precondition *together with the touch* for the ultimate experience as of two tactile objects. In any case, it is definitely not a logical precondition because no one who has never experienced Aristotle's illusions before would figure it out by sheer a priori reflection that when one's fingers are crossed and touched by one object, one must be in a proprioceptive state of awareness of one's fingers as uncrossed, and hence perceive the touch as if caused by two objects.

There are several versions of this illusion. One version brings about the reverse sensation, that of one object touching the fingers in between, when in fact there are two objects touched to the

[2]Let me note a few details. Of course, in a sense, even when we feel as if we are touched by two objects when our fingers are crossed, there is a component of our experience which indicates that the fingers are crossed, namely, the experience that is brought about by the stretch receptors of the skin and of the joints. Other receptors involved at the more global level of proprioception are the ones to be found in the muscles, more exactly at the level of muscle spindles. Plausibly enough, all these receptors still act on our consciousness, yet when the touch occurs, some of them go in the background and the tactile feeling of two objects dominates, so that ultimately it induces a proprioceptive illusion. That's why I consider it as a tactile-proprioceptive illusion, even though it sometimes appears under the heading of tactile illusions in the literature. In any case, the difference between our subjective states before and at the moment of touch is explained as a difference in proprioceptive states caused by a tactile stimulus. So I take this case as one that shows that sometimes proprioception depends on some tactile stimulus.

external sides of the crossed fingers (Rivers 1894). If you doubt that these are really cases of *proprioceptive* illusion, or that there could be proprioceptive illusions in general, then here is a more radical case, when a tactile stimulus coupled with a visual one brings about a situation in which (a) there clearly is an illusion, (b) it cannot be tactile, and (3) it cannot be visual, so it is clearly proprioceptive. It is a truly and radically novel experience resulting from two ordinary experiences, one visual and one tactile. Ehrsson (2009) describes an experiment[3] in which a combination of visual and tactile stimulation leads to a radically illusory proprioception of the body plan. The body plan of an organism is the most fundamental proprioceptive element, as it refers to the symmetry and the number of segments and limbs belonging to the organism and it imposes well-known fundamental constraints on the neural representations of the body. This fact is welcome by champions of the embodied cognition movement in recent cognitive science. However, there are illusions that occur even at the level of the body plan. Ehrsson's subjects were made to sit at a table, with the right hand hidden under it, and were presented in full view on the table with two prosthetic rubber arms with hands and fingers. The two rubber arms were touched simultaneously, in a sweeping motion, by two parallel brushes, on the index finger. Simultaneously with these brush sweeps the subject's hidden hand was touched by a brush in a synchronized way with the brush sweeps on the rubber hands. Ehrsson describes the resulting sensation as follows:

> After 2 min. of brushing, the majority of people tested reported sensing the paintbrushes on both rubber hands, i.e. they had two spatially distinct sensations of being touched, one on 'each'. People also often described how both rubber hands felt like their own right hand at the same time. (2009: 310)

What is really interesting about this experiment is that it brings about a proprioceptive state that is truly novel, first, because it is the result of stimuli that are proper to other sense modalities than proprioception (i.e., vision and touch), and, second, because it involves a radical restructuring of the very body plan (a sensation of having *two* right hands, and, as if that was not enough, neither of them happens to be the real one). It is also noteworthy that although we clearly have a massive illusion in this case, it is neither tactile, nor visual. The tactile sensation is veridical: the feeling of being

---

[3] A version of the well-known rubber hand illusion (Botvinick and Cohen 1998).

touched in a sweeping motion by a paintbrush. Similarly, the visual information is correct: two rubber hands being touched in a sweeping motion by two paintbrushes simultaneously. So we have a massive proprioceptive illusion caused by veridical non-proprioceptive stimuli.

This example also shows, maybe even more clearly than Aristotle's illusion, that it is not always the case that touch is logically and causally posterior to proprioception. In this case, like in the previous one, you simply can't predict the proprioceptive percept from the knowledge of the applied stimuli, so we can't assert that the proprioceptive percept of having two right arms and, moreover, both distinct from the real one, is logically presupposed in describing the tactile stimulus.

The main reason, however, for bringing up tactile-proprioceptive illusions is not to criticize O'Shaughnessy, but to use one such case as the basis for an argument for embodied consciousness, that is, an argument that in some cases the only option we have is to take the PNS processes associated with a conscious experience as constitutive of that experience, and not causing that experience. To my knowledge, neither the illusion I will describe (a version of the Aristotle illusion), nor the argument that I will construct have been presented and discussed before, in either philosophy, or the neuroscience and cognitive psychology literature. Indeed, Fabrizio Benedetti, cited before for his seminal contributions in the neuroscience of tactile and tactile-proprioceptive illusions, confirmed in personal correspondence that the illusion I have discovered while experimenting on myself with the original Aristotle's illusion has not previously been described in the literature, or at least not the way I do.[4]

What I do is the following. I lie down on my back and keep my left palm perpendicular with respect to my body, a few centimeters above it, with the thumb pointing towards the body, and with fingers 1 (index) and 2 (middle) crossed (finger 2 above finger 1). Then I touch, say, finger 2 first and then finger 1 with a pencil. To do this, I intend and move the pencil upwards, but when it makes the second touch, namely on finger 1, the movement feels as if it was not upwards but downwards. So the experience of the direction in which I move the pencil feels both upwards and downwards roughly at the

---

[4]Later I found something close to this illusion in a brief note in the very first issue of *Mind*, by G. C. Robertson (1876: 145–46). However, he does not focus on the aspects of it that I found important as a basis for the embodied mind hypothesis and does not offer a causal analysis of the type I do here of what is going on. However, many points I will make have also been stated by Robertson.

same time, that is, if we take the whole time stretch between the two contacts as an atomic interval to correspond to the total motion we execute. It is a paradoxical feeling. I go upwards, so I expect to touch the finger that is above, and yet I end up touching the finger that feels below. So it is like a tactile version of Escher's ascending-descending staircase. Of course, mutatis mutandis for: (a) touching sequence from above to below, and (b) the palm's changed orientation, with thumb up. It works best when I don't look at the fingers.

Let us see what is going on in this case. First, let us break the total experience down into two components. One component is the experience at the level of the left hand, with fingers crossed. The other component is at the level of the right hand, whose finger is used as the moving, active tactile stimulus. What we are interested in regarding the first part of the experience is tactile sensing, whereas with respect to the second part we focus on kinesthesia, that is, the sense of motion of the finger.[5] As already noted by Robertson (1876), when moving the finger, say, upwards, and hitting the finger on its way, it feels at the level of the crossed fingers that the finger has been hit from below, although in reality that finger is above (i.e., the index finger), because it is crossed with the next one (i.e., the middle finger). Robertson only focused on this phenomenon and speculated, correctly, that this means that there are regions on our skin that are intrinsically felt as located, namely, relative to other regions on the skin.[6] I agree with this point, and I will call the distance between the fingertips, either measured between their interiors or between their exteriors, when the fingers are not crossed, the *intrinsic proprioceptive phenomenal distance* (IPPD). On the other hand, I will refer to the physical distance between the fingertips the *extrinsic exteroceptive distance* (EED). Related to these there are also two notions of orientation of the finger: *intrinsic proprioceptive phenomenal orientation* (IPPO) and *extrinsic exteroceptive orientation* (EEO). These orientations take two values: interiors and exteriors. Hence we have

[5] Of course, the moving finger also receives tactile information due to the contacts with the fingers on the other hand, but it is intuitively irrelevant to take it into consideration, so we can safely neglect it.

[6] Since Robertson's insight, several authors (e.g., Merleau-Ponty [1995] 2003, [1945] 2002; O'Shaughnessy 1995; Gallagher 2003) have made the more general point that the spatial frame of proprioception is special in that it is not relative to anything outside itself. For instance, in vision spatial relations, like "being to the right," involve relativity to the position of one's body, hence the predicate is dyadic, but in the case of proprioception this predicate is most naturally taken as monadic, so that ultimately proprioceptive location is not, either explicitly or implicitly, relative.

four types of orientation, all in all: *intrinsic proprioceptive phenomenal interior (IPPI), intrinsic proprioceptive phenomenal exterior (IPPE), extrinsic exteroceptive interior (EEI),* and *extrinsic exteroceptive exterior (EEE).* What happens in the double tactile sensation case, when the fingers are crossed, is that while the IPPDs and IPPOs between the interiors and between the exteriors remain intact through the finger crossing, because they are intrinsic, the EEDs and EEOs change, as they are extrinsic. The result of the change is that now the EED between the exteriors is as small as the IPPD between the interiors and their EEOs are inward looking (so the exteriors face each other rather than facing outwards) while the IPPD between the exteriors stays constant and is therefore felt as a large distance. Since the large IPPD between the exteriors is correlated with the phenomenon of being touched simultaneously by two objects, and never by one, because the IPPOs are contrary to each other and outward looking, the touch will be felt as if coming from two objects, when the fingers get crossed (figure 7.2).

However, I would like to move beyond this level and consider what happens within the other component of the total experience, the one related to the proprioception of the active tactile stimulus, the moving index finger of the right hand. As I have mentioned before, when describing the Escher type proprioceptive experience of the successive touch of crossed fingers (see the details of the setup before), when we move our finger upwards, from the intrinsic exterior of the middle finger to the intrinsic exterior of the index finger, the movement feels both upwards and downwards once the second touch occurs. This experience is a distinct component from the experience at the level of the hand with crossed fingers, though it depends on it. This experience also constitutes a good basis to formulate my argument for the constitutive contribution of the PNS.

Let us consider the experience itself of the motion of the finger being both upwards and downwards (or if your hand is in a vertical position: both to the left and to the right[7]), and its potential causal relation to what happens at the level of the PNS of the other hand. Whether the peripheral touch and proprioception sensors at the level of the crossed fingers have a *causal* contribution to some component

---

[7] As Benedetti notes, in private communication, the same paradoxical vertical versus horizontal illusory movement can be obtained by displacing other body parts by 90 degrees. For example, try with your lips: you can place your lower lip in different positions relative to the upper lip and you will experience many interesting illusory movement directions, doubling of objects, doubling of lines, and such like.

IPPE   EEI

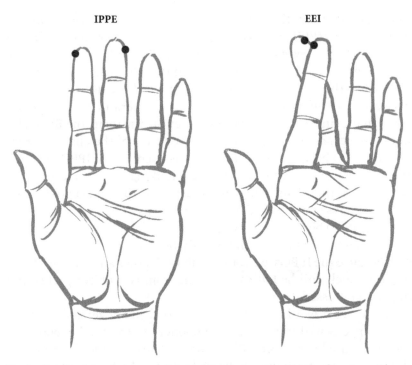

Figure 7.2 Position in space of the intrinsic interiors of the fingers, with normal and crossed fingers. By crossing the fingers, Intrinsic Proprioceptive Phenomenal Exteriors (IPPE) become Extrinsic Exteroceptive Interiors (EEI).

of the Escher type experience we could figure out by focusing on certain counterfactuals having that experiential component as consequent, and some PNS facts as antecedent.[8] Let us consider the first such counterfactual, assuming that we moved our active finger upwards, and focus on the appearance of the motion as being downwards, set this latter component as our consequent:

> (A) Had the fingers not been crossed, everything else being equal, the upward motion of the active finger would not have been also felt as downward.

---

[8]If one is skeptical that the counterfactual analysis of causation is good enough and thinks that the counterfactual conditional being false is not sufficient for proving the lack of causal contribution, it is worth pointing out that the only counterexamples to the necessity of a counterfactual dependence of effect on cause are ones in which the counterfactuals are false because there is some backup cause that would get activated if the cause event were not present. But our case is not like that; there is no backup cause anywhere in the background to intervene in case the finger crossing does not occur.

Whether this counterfactual is true depends on what is held fixed in virtue of the clause "everything else being equal." Let us notice first that not everything *can* be equal if we are to keep the counterfactual situation within the bounds of the nomologically possible. For example, we can't keep the order of the two touches relative to the intrinsic orientations of the fingertips constant, namely, from the intrinsic exterior of the middle finger to the intrinsic exterior of the index finger, and execute this motion upwards, unless we have a very curved space such that a motion upwards will end up hitting the index finger from below.

In the first case, let us hold the intrinsic origin and destination of the touch constant. Counterfactual (A) is false because, as explained above, the required motion is nomologically constrained to proceed downwards. In the second case, we hold the extrinsic origin and destination fixed, namely, we are required to proceed from the extrinsic interior of whichever finger is extrinsically below to the extrinsic interior of whichever finger is extrinsically above. In this second case, the counterfactual is true because the motion is both objectively and subjectively only upwards. However, the reason the counterfactual is true in this second case is because by uncrossing the fingers the intrinsic interiors become again extrinsic interiors as well, while the regions that used to be the extrinsic interiors when the fingers were crossed are now intrinsic and extrinsic exteriors, so the successive touches by the active finger will proceed from the intrinsic interior of the index finger (which is now both felt as and physically lower) to the intrinsic interior of the middle finger (which is now both felt as and physically higher). This means that the more fundamental counterfactual, in virtue of which (A) is true under this second interpretation of what is held fixed, is the following:

> (B) Had the extrinsic interiors of the fingers not been intrinsic exteriors, everything else being equal, the upward motion of the active finger would not have been also felt as downward.

However, empirical research shows (Benedetti 1991) that when human subjects are exposed to long-lasting tactile reversal (six months in Benedetti's experiment), their tactile perception ceases to be illusory, that is, after they have their fingers crossed for a long time, they cease to have the Aristotle illusion or any version of it. Their motor response and perception are all correct when with fingers crossed. Furthermore, Benedetti proves his "extended range hypothesis," according to which after variable time with fingers crossed the perceptual system extends in terms of the functional range of the fingers when they are crossed, rather than a mere adaptation taking place, by which the perceptual system loses its capacities when fingers are uncrossed. This is proven by the fact that after long-term finger crossing subjects do not lose their motor and perceptual abilities when fingers are not crossed. In other words, after long-term reversal, whether the fingers are crossed or not does not matter; the subjects are equally good at identifying and perceiving objects correctly with crossed and with uncrossed fingers. Finally, Benedetti also shows that when a trained (i.e., crossed for a long time) finger gets crossed with an untrained one (one that has not yet been crossed with any other finger for long enough time) the same tactile illusions occur, which means that pairs of crossed fingers form independent perceptual systems at the level of the hand.

What I want to derive from here as a conclusion is that whether a region on the fingertip is an intrinsic interior and whether its intrinsic orientation is downward or upward (in the setup I described in my own Escher type experiment) does not depend on whether fingers are crossed or not at a particular time, but rather on whether those regions have a history of having received sufficient stimulation from the external tactile objects. A fact about our world is that we rarely receive tactile stimulation that is simultaneous on the exterior sides of the fingers. Such objects are rare and such stimulation is most likely to occur in artificial setting and with very complex voluntarily controlled human actions as the source of the stimulation. On the other hand, the daily exploration of the environment brings about a lot of stimulation of the interior sides of the fingers, for example, when holding a cigarette between the fingers, or when writing with a pen, and many others. So, as a matter of fact, the real cause of the Escher type motion illusion when I cross my fingers for the first time is an absence; the absence of a sufficiently long stimulation of the touch contacts.[9] But the absence of such a history of stimulation is not the type of process that is present at the level of the contact points of the touch when I do have the illusion. The lack of stimulation is not a positive fact about the PNS when I am touched. So the positive fact about the PNS when I am touched, namely, that the nerve endings become activated, is not a causal

---

[9]This point is congenial to Gibson's hypothesis about perception as an information pick-up system or a system that works as a matter of tuning to information, where "information" refers to objective environmental invariances, and to Gibson's point that the perceiver is a self-tuning system (1966: 271, 1979: 248–50)

contributor to my experience, since the only one causal contributor, if we follow the counterfactual analysis, is the lack of sufficient past stimulation. Yet, it is pretty clear that the one-shot stimulation of those contacts, when I cross the fingers, is a contributor to my paradoxical experience. So we should understand these PNS processes as constitutive contributors to the experience.

Let me make a brief analogy here, which will show how to intuitively separate the causal components from the constitutive components. To change the famous story a bit, the Count of Monte Cristo, who is trapped in his prison cell, follows the Mad Priest's escape plan, and they start digging a tunnel through the thick stone walls of the prison fortress, having their spoons as their only usable tool. They need to dig for ten years in order to complete the five-meter-long hole that would enable them to escape. Suppose we focus on the hole as it appears after five years of digging. Suppose the Mad Priest scrapes out half a spoonful of detritus from the wall. The scraping of the wall is a cause of the hole becoming, say, two meters long, but, intuitively, why they are still trapped is because there has not been sufficient scraping yet. The absence of sufficient scraping is the cause of their being trapped. But what about the hole being two meters long? Intuitively, this is not a cause of their being trapped, but a constituent of this fact. To be trapped, in that situation, is partly constituted by the fact that the hole is not five meters long yet. Similarly, when the hole becomes five meters long, that fact will constitute their escape, although the hole becoming that long was caused by the constant scraping for ten years. The scraping is a cause of the escape, but the length of the hole constitutes it. You can now replace the lengthy successive scraping above with the lengthy successive stimulation of the finger skin by external surfaces, and the length of the hole with the current activity of the PNS at the level of the fingers, and you get the way I think of the PNS as constitutive of the experience.

Finally, let me address a detail about why I appealed to my version of the tactile-proprioceptive illusion, the Escher type up-down sensation of finger movement. The standard Aristotle's illusion would bring about the same results of a causal analysis, but I think my version is better for two reasons. The first reason is that the experience is clearly paradoxical, as it is contradictory; it contains motion that is felt to proceed both upward and downward. This demands an explanation, so we are less tempted to explain the experience away, or to argue that there is nothing really illusory about it, as one might be tempted to could argue in the classic Aristotle's illusion. The second reason is that, unlike in Aristotle's illusion, the felt experience of motion is clearly partly at the level of the active finger, the one we use for touching the crossed fingers, and not exclusively at the level of the passive, crossed fingers. Again, this adds to the air of paradoxicality of the experience and also offers a good example of how proprioceptively clearly separate regions of the body (left hand versus right hand) become a phenomenal unit by their action upon one another.

II. *Phenomenal Embodiment and Proprioceptive Innervation*

There are several questions that one could raise when it comes to the issue of how the body is related to the mind. One such question is whether the body is merely *represented* by the mind, as in a body image, or is a constitutive part of what the mind is or does. There has been a long tradition of conceptual confusion related to these two ways in which the body could be present to the mind, namely, both scientists and the few philosophers who were interested in a more active role of the body in the mind used to talk of body image and body schema interchangeably. Shaun Gallagher (2005: ch. 1) offers a nice historical and philosophical overview of this confusion.[10] As pointed out in chapter 1, what I am ultimately interested in is not as much the notion of a body image, or how the brain consciously represents the body in its various states (i.e., the body-in-the-brain). Rather, the more interesting and more basic notion from the point of view of this book is the notion of "body schema," which is not a conscious representation of the body, or of the bodily states, but an unconscious and always present constraint on what the mind can do. What I try in this context to bring in as an item for our analytical focus is the role of the PNS, in order to move beyond the general notion of "body."

Following Gallagher (2005), we can point out several differences between the body image and the body schema. One is that whereas the body image contains body percepts, which I come to instantiate in virtue of consciously attending to my own body, the body schema is always in excess of what can be consciously attended to. For instance, even when I focus on my body's posture and movement, so these aspects of my body become part of my body image at that

---

[10] See also Gallagher 2012, for a defense of the distinction, as a reply to Berlucchi and Aglioti 2010.

time, the body schema continues to function unconsciously, enabling my balance and movement. Second, whereas the body image involves the sense of ownership, which is a person-level conscious experience, the body schema can function autonomously even when certain parts of the body are not perceived as belonging to oneself. Third, the body image is based on attention, and so it will always involve a partial representation of the body, whereas the body schema involves a global and all-encompassing integrated system. Fourth, the body schema can involve parts of the environment, external to the body, which otherwise the body image would not allow to become part of it. The previously described case of proprioceptive doubling of the right arm is such a case.

However, to say that the body schema does an unconscious enabling job does not mean that it is disconnected or functioning totally autonomously from the experience of one's body. I would like in what follows to focus on certain cases of what I call "primal body image," which I take as cases in which a part of the body image constitutively involves processes that form the body schema.[11]

The reason I talk about "a part of the body image" is that the notion of a body image is very general, and it involves not only conscious proprioceptive experiences but also highly abstract beliefs about one's body, desires and imaginings involving one's body, and all the possible types of exteroceptive awareness of one's body. This means, in my view, that the notion of body image per se does not prove very useful from the point of view of the analysis of experience, as it is quite gerrymandered. Nevertheless, let us first set up a distinction among various types of being aware of or attending to one's body, which will prove useful later in this section, when I will argue against the "ultra-Cartesian," but still orthodox among philosophers, view that one's disembodiment is logically possible or imaginable.

---

[11] An anonymous referee has expressed skepticism about the very notion of body schema, claiming that the difference between this and the body itself is hard to see. As I see it, the difference is that the body schema is supposed to be understood as an information pool (where information is understood in the Gibsonian way, as a set of items in the environment, here 'environment' being the body itself), whereas the body as such is understood independently of what information it provides to the nervous system. So the very same bodily property might be considered as a source of information versus independently of what information it generates. For instance, consider the bodily property of having lower limbs of unequal lengths. Taken merely as a property of some body as such, it is about some lengths of some material parts and the relation between them. But taken as part of the body schema, this property of the body is about the constraints it places on, e.g., kinesthesia.

There are various ways in which we could be aware of our body, and we can arrange them on a scale from less intimate, through more intimate, to self-awareness as such. First, we can be or become aware of our body without being aware whatsoever that it is our body. These are cases of *exteroceptive awareness of one's body not qua one's own body*. This case could be further divided into one in which we positively perceive our body as not being our own, as being alien, like in Body Image Identity Disorder, and one in which we merely fail to notice that the body we are aware of is our own, like when we perceive part of our body in a mirror, failing to notice that what we see is a mirror reflection of a body part of our own. The second category is represented by cases of *exteroceptive awareness of one's body qua one's own body*. Obviously, these are cases of more intimate connection between us and what we are aware of. For instance, looking at our limbs, touching our own face, and so on are such cases. Finally, there are cases of *proprioceptive awareness of one's body*. This last phrase is in fact pleonastic, as one cannot proprioceive anything but one's own body (see below for a discussion), and for that reason one also cannot proprioceive one's body otherwise than qua one's own. Proprioception is in this sense a form of self-awareness, and the notion of ownership in the expression "I proprioceive my body" is really a form of identity. This is in my view the right notion of proprioception proper, rather than any notion that makes it similar to exteroception. For instance, again, O'Shaughnessy seems to equate proprioception with some bodily version of exteroception:

> Why not abandon the theory of a body-directed attending, and substitute in its place an account in which we postulate an immediate knowledge of limb presence and posture which is generated by psycho-cerebral phenomena regularly caused by such bodily states of affairs? I am convinced that this would be a mistake. To help explain why, I will begin this examination of proprioception by considering an atypical example of the species. Namely, the case in which we involve some of our perceptual attention away from its usual visual and auditory objects, and actively turn it instead in an immediate mode onto some body part like an arm. This is an atypical example of proprioception, partly because of its purely inquisitive character, but above all because it draws its object out of its natural obscurity into the full light of awareness. Yet I doubt whether it differs much from the everyday recessive examples in other significant respects. In any case, it is surely an example of perception. (2000: 628–29)

As a matter of fact, I think that what O'Shaughnessy refers to as an atypical case of proprioception is not really proprioception. Try to attend to some body part of yours, *proprioceptively*. Probably the easiest to do is to flex some muscle, say, in the leg and then attend to how it feels. What I end up with while doing this is just trying to focus on what I feel, or what my muscle experience is like, which, in other words, is the same as introspecting. Introspection, I take it, is not a form of proprioception, but of exteroception. It involves rather figuring out and becoming aware of how it feels "up here," so to say, whatever is happening "down there." Proprioception proper, at least in my view, is rather "silently being down there." Proprioception is a silent sense, by which I mean that it is not supposed to involve (and, in fact, it is supposed to *exclude*) any effort of attending, focusing, expecting. Introspection is closer to standard exteroception, like vision or hearing, in that it involves the perceiving self in relation to something outside itself, even if this sounds paradoxical. It only sounds paradoxical because the intentional object of introspection is itself a vehicle with its own intentional object. But the difference, from the point of view of comparing introspection with proprioception, is not essential: whereas in visual perception an external object appears to the perceiving self some way or other, in introspection an internal object, or rather state, appears to the perceiving self some way or other. In contrast, in proprioception there is nothing like an object to appear some way or other, but rather the self or mind suffusing the body in all its parts that are properly innervated (i.e., containing intact and normally functioning proprioceptive receptors and nerve fibers).

We can also look at the same things from an opposite perspective, as it were, namely, from the felt proximity of the objects that various sense modalities make us represent. Although philosophers have been talking about the intentional object of perception, implicitly supposing that there is such a unitary notion that can be generalized over all sense modalities, in my view we can clearly rank these objects in terms of their phenomenal or felt proximity to us. This felt proximity has to do, if I am right, with the extent of phenomenal presence of the self at the periphery that is the proper receptor associated with each intentional object in perception. Thus, vision seems to me at one extreme, in that it loses us to the world. When you visually perceive some object, no matter whether it is far or close, you are completely unaware of the PNS processes that, if I am right, partly constitute your visual percepts. In chapter 2, I presented and discussed the debates within neuroscience about whether we are "directly aware of our retina." Now, it looks to me that, to begin with, those neuroscientists misuse the notion of being aware of.

They, of course, don't really mean what they say when formulating the question of the debate that way; I suppose it is simply a way to simplify vocabulary. However, in philosophy we are not supposed to use the terms so loosely. So when I say that in vision we are unaware of the PNS processes at the level of the eye, this is also true for any other part of the nervous system, including the brain. Of course, when we look at and see an object, we are aware of that object, and not of anything going on in our nervous system. Too bad for neuroscientists who talk of "being aware of cortical area such-and-such." The question in neuroscience should more correctly be stated as: What are the neural processes that realize the awareness of a visual object? So, what I say is that in vision we are typically aware of an external reality *without remainder*. In other words, the object that is felt as external exhausts everything we are aware of. Things are similar with most other exteroceptive sense modalities. Hearing a sound, except in cases when it is dominated by bone-conduction, is not felt as internal in any way.[12] Of course, some supraliminal sound stimulus can cause vibration in the inner ear felt via mechanoception (i.e., felt as mechanical vibration proper), in which case we become aware of some process that is felt as being at the level of the ear. However, such cases are not cases of hearing as such, but hearing plus mechanoception, a form of tactile perception. The sense of smell, again with the exception of retronasal olfaction,[13] is somehow in between as far as the felt proximity of its intentional object is concerned, not only because, as some authors have pointed out (Peacocke 1983; Lycan 2000; Batty 2010), there does not seem to exist any intentional object proper in the case of smell as compared to vision, which makes the felt smell more subjective or mind-dependent, but also because felt proximity depends on some qualities of the particular smell one is experiencing. For instance, when one is driving in the countryside and passes by a pig farm, the strong smell is felt as close, in the car,

---

[12] A case of hearing that presents the sound as internal is the case of food sounds when processed in the mouth. When chewing occurs with the mouth closed, we hear this sound as internal. Another case is the sound of your nervous system; thus, composer John Cage confesses his revelation when entering an anechoic chamber (a special room with no echo, informally called "silent room") when he "heard two sounds, one high and one low. When I described them to the engineer in charge, he informed me that the high one was my nervous system in operation, the low one my blood in circulation" (Cage [1939] 1961: 8). In all such cases the sound is bone-conducted rather than air-conducted.

[13] Retronasal olfaction plays a crucial role in flavor perception, and unlike orthonasal olfaction, which requires inspiration of air through the nose, it is generated via expiration of air through the nose. See Rozin 1982.

if not downright in one's nose, whereas a slight smell of freshly baked bread is felt as coming from somewhere, rather than being in one's nose. Of course, there are higher cognitive (belief that the smell is coming from somewhere) and emotional (desire that it came from farther or from closer, depending on whether it is felt as offensive or pleasant) components that are responsible for these differences, and probably the main variable responsible for the tendency to feel a smell close or far is the intensity; when the smell is less intense, it tends to be felt as farther, and vice versa.

The sense of touch is the one that brings its intentional objects phenomenally the closest to the experiencing subject, while keeping that object phenomenally distinct from or external to the mind. In normal cases of both active touch (i.e., touching) and passive touch (i.e., being touched), the tactile external object is felt as making a contact with us. There is no intervening phenomenal presence of anything else, that is, of an intentional object based on anything else than either touch or proprioception.

Finally, proprioception and interoception are senses whose intentional objects are not distinguished from our experiencing self. I have already discussed proprioception, but interoception has only been briefly mentioned before, although pain, which some authors have more recently argued that it should be considered a form of interoception (Craig 2003), has also been extensively discussed in chapter 3. Interoception is the system that brings about sensations associated with visceral and other internal signals. Some examples are hunger, thirst, vasomotor activity, and if the more recent arguments for reconceptualization are right, then pain, temperature, and itch would also count as such. From the point of view of the phenomenal closeness of its intentional object, interoception seems to me at the other extreme from vision. Interoceptive qualia, though sometimes highly indistinct and structureless, seem to clearly be felt inside oneself, and, unlike in (soft) touch, not in a way that phenomenally distinguishes the self from the world outside. Also, unlike proprioception, interoception is typically not a silent sense; its states are present only when they are brought into attentional awareness, like in the case of hunger or thirst. It looks like whereas visual phenomenology brings about losing oneself to the external world, interoceptive phenomenology brings about losing oneself to some internal location of oneself. As about pain and especially temperature, these sensations have, in my opinion, both an exteroceptive and an interoceptive phenomenology, and which of these two subjective aspects prevails depends on the specific stimulus.

Let us return then to proprioception. As I have said a few paragraphs above, in proprioception there is nothing like an object to
appear some way or other, but rather the self or mind suffusing the
body in all its parts that contain intact proprioceptive receptors and
nerve fibers. It is, of course, artificial to separate all these senses and
types of sensations when it comes to real experiences, where there
is a complex interplay among several of them. The phenomenology
of one's having a body of one's own, or of one being present every-
where in one's body, which I call the "primal body image" is a matter of interplay among proprioception, tactile perception, and
interoception. What is responsible for this feeling of being embodied, or rather the body being "enminded" is the PNS, and according
to the main thesis proposed in this book, in a constitutive way. One
could well be skeptical about this allegedly constitutive relation
between innervation and the bodily presence of the self. For instance,
cases of phantom limb pain, or cases like the one I have discussed,
the illusory phenomenal doubling and incarnation into two rubber
arms of one's felt right arm, show that one can feel one's body extend
to regions that are not innervated whatsoever. Here is the same
problem considered and answered by Merleau-Ponty, who, like me
here, does find the peripheral mind hypothesis congenial:

> Thus exteroceptivity demands that stimuli be given a shape; the con-
> sciousness of the body invades the body, the soul spreads over all its
> parts, and behavior overspills its central sector. But one might reply
> that this "bodily experience" is itself a representation, a "psychic fact,"
> and that as such it is at the end of a chain of physical and physiological
> events which alone can be ascribed to the real body.... Is it then neces-
> sary to abandon the "peripheral theory" in favor of a "central theory"?
> But a central theory would get us no further if it added no more to the
> peripheral conditions of the imaginary limb than cerebral symptoms.
> For a collection of cerebral symptoms could not represent the relation-
> ships in consciousness which enter the phenomenon. It depends indeed
> on "psychic" determinants." An emotion, circumstance which recalls
> those in which the wound was received, creates a phantom limb in
> subjects who had none.... Must we then conclude that the phantom
> limb is a memory, a volition or a belief, and, failing any physiological
> explanation, must we provide a psychological explanation for it? *But no
> psychological explanation can overlook the fact that the severance of
> the nerves to the brain abolishes the phantom limb.* ([1945] 2002:
> 88–89) (emphasis added)

What Merleau-Ponty points out in his reply to the "central theory"
is that cases like the phantom limb do not show that the PNS is not

important, witness that total deafferentation (cutting off the afferent peripheral nerves from neck down) makes the phantom limb disappear. So it is not as if the phantom limb by itself shows that the PNS is disposable when it comes to explaining and ontically basing the phenomenology. The closest we can get to a case in which the phantom limb could falsify my hypothesis and reinforce the central theory is discussed in recent neuroscience in connection with phantom limb sensations in patients with congenitally missing limbs. These phantoms are interesting in that the patients have never had any limb in their lives, so it is puzzling how these vivid phantom limb sensations arise. However, even in these cases the explanation neuroscientists have recently come up with is that the phantom is a result of "the monitoring of reafference signals derived from the motor commands sent to the phantom during gesticulation" (Ramachandran and Hirstein 1998: 1606), which means, if I have understood it correctly, that ultimately the phantom sensation requires reafference signals, that is some PNS components.[14]

As it was apparent in chapter 3, when I discussed the Gate Control Theory of Pain, pain sensations are many times based on random signals in regions of the PNS that are not represented by the sensation itself. Similarly, in cases of peripheral nerve damage there is hyperalgesia although strictly speaking there are fewer nerves as a result of the damage. When I had my peripheral nerve damage, I was initially puzzled as to why I felt quite intense pain when pressure was applied to certain areas on my legs, given that (i) my damage was overwhelmingly motor, not sensory, and (ii) anyway, intuitively, chemical or mechanical damage to the *nerves themselves* should not hurt, as they are not self-sensitive.[15] I used to feel pain when having my legs crossed for more than a minute or so, which was the result of pressure on the lateral part of the crossed leg, where the *medial sural cutaneous nerve* is located, which is itself a branch of the *sciatic nerve*—the longest and widest nerve fiber in the human body. I was not familiar at the time with anything about the neuroscience of pain, so no wonder I was puzzled by this pain. What

---

[14] Reafference is the sensory feedback the source of which is one's own motor action or series of motor actions.

[15] People sometimes express amazement that the brain, which is the "center for pain," is not itself sensitive to noxious stimuli applied mechanically to it. But the same is true of any typical individual neuron and any typical individual nerve fiber of the PNS: they are supposed to capture the noxious stimulus via the chemical neurotransmitters at their dendritic terminations, and not by being sectioned or chemically destroyed.

happens, however, is that when peripheral damage occurs, there is typically a process called "peripheral sensitization," which generates hypersensitivity in certain parts of the PNS, which are *not* themselves damaged. To keep to my particular autobiographical example, painful sensitivity to medium pressure applied to the sural nerve occurs shortly after damage to other parts of the sciatic nerve. According to the animal model proposed by Decosterd and Woolf (2000), the spared nerve injury model, a lesion of two of the three terminal branches of the sciatic nerve—*tibial* and *common peroneal* nerves—leaving the remaining sural nerve intact, results in early (i.e., within less than twenty-four hours), robust (i.e., occurs in virtually all denervated animals), and prolonged (i.e., more than six months) pain-specific behavioral changes related to stimulation of intact skin areas innervated by the sural.

There is no reason not to think of the above-mentioned illusory proprioceptive experiences on this model, that is, as still dependent in a constitutive manner on some PNS activity, even if not always in a non-illusory way.

To conclude this section, we feel ourselves not *in a body*, but *as a body*. Proprioception, interoception, and touch interact in ways to create this "enminded body" experience, and it is not implausible, illusory experiences notwithstanding, that this presence in all parts of the body essentially involves intact PNS innervation of many parts of the body, given that complete afferent peripheral denervation results in no such proprioceptive experience, not even in illusory ones.

III. *Against Proper Disembodiment*

Many philosophers, especially antinaturalists (e.g., Descartes), but also some materialists of an older school (e.g., Armstrong [1968] 2002: 19) are fond of the logical possibility of disembodiment, that is, the logical possibility that one, or one's mind, could exist without a material body whatsoever. There is a quite extensive literature on this problem and its ramifications, but it seems to me that certain further questions and subtleties that arise have not been properly addressed, and that the disembodiment claim has been left at this, in my view, rough state, as expressed in the previous sentence.

I want to know more about what exactly is claimed when someone claims that it is logically possible that I, as the mind that I am, be disembodied. We can raise questions and try to further clarify what is involved in the scenario of a disembodied mind on two fronts: on the side of the mind and on that of the body. I will start with the latter.

What is meant by "body" when it comes to the thing that the disembodied mind should lack? How far is the state of bodilessness from the state of embodied existence, as far as what is lacking in the latter is concerned? Here we can focus on three general aspects of our bodies with respect to which the bodiless mind's state could be compared: morphology, structure, and function. At one extreme we have a bodiless mind in the sense that there is nothing morphologically, structurally, and functionally similar to our bodies that this mind is embedded into. I will call this type of mind "pure angel" or, alternatively, "perfect ghost." What the pure angel is embedded into is nothing whatsoever, not even air or some otherworldly gas.

Then we have a mind which is not embodied in a body like ours, but in something else, say, angelic matter, ghost stuff, ectoplasm, aura, ethereal body, or some such, which we can call "quasi-body." It is incorporeal in the weaker sense than the pure angel, it is *ethereal*. Such quasi-bodies are, to be sure, morphologically different from our bodies; I reckon they are supposed not to be solid, not to have shape and mechanical properties like our bodies have, and also be unavailable to our senses, except probably under special circumstances and when the mind wills them to be detected. Nevertheless these quasi-bodies are closer to our actual bodies than the minds with no bodylike entity at all to support them, that is, the pure angels. Suppose also that these quasi-bodies are amorphous (structureless) and their ethereal parts or regions fulfill no function. Let us call the minds embedded in this kind of a body "stuffy angels" or "dull ghosts." It is then a further addition to their powers if they possess some structure and function such that they can respond and intervene in the ongoings of the physical world around them. This third type of minded quasi-body is then morphologically, structurally, and functionally, similar to the minded bodies that we are. For better or for worse, I will call the minds that are disembodied in this sense "vulgar angels," or, following my own earlier terminology (Aranyosi 2007), "Hollywood ghosts."

In terms of how interesting they are from an external point of view, the pure angel/perfect ghost is least so; it is so pure/perfect that it is logically guaranteed that it will never come to bring you some divine message/haunt your house, or make itself ever detectable in any way. The stuffy angel/dull ghost is detectable when it wills so; it will be able to play the Poltergeist, to make itself felt by radiating or by spreading some smell or "psychic energy" (Hart 1988) and so on. Finally, the vulgar angel/Hollywood ghost will behave and exert causal influence in complex enough ways, according as what the specific situation requires; think about the messenger role of the angels in the Hebrew and Christian Bibles and in the Qur'an, or about the ghost in the Hollywood movie *Ghost*.

The other side from which we can approach and clarify what is meant by disembodiment is the side of the mind. If previously our question was how much of the actual body is going to be missing in the disembodiment scenario, the question we can ask now is: How much of the actual mind is going to be *preserved* in conceivable cases of mind without body? In other words, how close to our minds will the conceived disembodied one be?

Again, at one extreme we will have a copy of the totality of our own mental states, in all their richness and intricacy. Let's call such a mind "realistic mind." At an intermediate level the disembodied mind will only be a copy of one simple enough mental state, for instance, a short pain state with the afferent emotional and cognitive components, and nothing else. I will call this type of disembodied mind "simple mind." Finally, at the other extreme we have a disembodied mind that only copies one single aspect of one of our experiences, for instance, a brief flash of experienced redness, with no emotional or cognitive components at all. This type I will call "dumb mind." Following the recipe I used in the case of types of bodies that disembodiment could be compatible with, let's call the types of disembodied minds that are less than realistic "quasi-minds."

Now we should join the two aspects of the disembodiment scenario, the body and the mind aspects, and see what kind of beings we can end up with having conceived. I want to argue that the more mind you want to disembody, the more body you will have to pack in, or, to express it using our terminology, the more realistic a disembodied mind is conceived to be, the more vulgar the angel (the more Hollywood the ghost) you end up with in the conceived scenario, so, in the extreme, you will not have succeeded in truly disembodying that mind; conversely, the purer the angel (the closer to perfection the ghost) you conceive of, the dumber it will be, so, in the extreme, you will not have succeeded in disembodying a true mind.

Let me first put one scenario off the table, as it might be confused with that of disembodiment in the relevant sense, and it should not. There is a sense of "mind without body," in which all of your current, past, and future experience is compatible with the nonexistence of anything in your environment. It is this sense which fuels the skeptical scenarios of various kinds, according to which, for all you know, the external world does not exist. And it is the same sense that fuels idealism, the view that identifies the apparently material world with a totality of experiences or collections of phenomenal particulars. That this sense of "mind without body" is irrelevant to our discussion can be made apparent by noticing that if disembodiment is claimed to be logically possible merely in this sense, then it has nothing to do especially with bodiless minds because in this sense everything is bodiless anyway, *including bodies themselves*, if by "body" we mean a material entity. Second, in this sense of disembodiment we might already actually be disembodied, for all we know.

The relevant sense of disembodiment is apparent if we focus on some quotes from Descartes, on the dualist side, and Armstrong, on the materialist side. Let's start with Armstrong, as it is self-explanatory:

> But disembodied existence seems to be a perfectly intelligible supposition. It may be that a good deal of perception presupposes that we have a body or at least a position in space. For instance, we see things as oriented in space with respect to *us*, and it is hard to see what 'us' refers to here if not to our body. But consider the case where I'm lying in bed at night thinking. Surely it is logically possible that I might be having just the same experiences, and yet not have a body at all? No doubt I am having certain somatic, that is to say, bodily, sensations. But if I am lying still these will not be very detailed in nature and I can see nothing self-contradictory in supposing that they do not correspond to anything in physical reality. Yet I need be in no doubt about my identity. ([1968] 2002: 19)

If what is meant by disembodiment were cases where our experiences, *no matter which*, could be the same as they actually are without there being any physical body at all, then Armstrong would not have bothered finding a case like when one is lying in bed thinking. He could have just taken any experience whatsoever, including bodily sensations, and say that they could be disembodied.

Next, Descartes, well before Armstrong, makes the same points about (i) bodily sensation as not relevant when one has to consider the possibility of disembodiment, and (ii) mere self-consciousness or thinking as the paradigm example of what is clearly possible to be disembodied. Thus in part 13 of *Meditation* 6, he supports the above point (i):

> Nature likewise teaches me by these sensations of pain, hunger, thirst, etc., that I am not only lodged in my body as a pilot in a vessel, but that I am besides so intimately conjoined, and as it were intermixed with it, that my mind and body compose a certain unity. For if this were not the case, I should not feel pain when my body is hurt, seeing I am merely a thinking thing, but should perceive the wound by the understanding alone, just as a pilot perceives by sight when any part of his vessel is damaged; and when my body has need of food or drink, I should have a clear knowledge of this, and not be made aware of it by the confused sensations of hunger and thirst: for, in truth, all these sensations of hunger, thirst, pain, etc., are nothing more than certain confused modes of thinking, arising from the union and apparent fusion of mind and body.

And in part 9 of the same mediation he considers and argues for point (ii) above:

> merely because I know with certitude that I exist, and because, in the meantime, I do not observe that aught necessarily belongs to my nature or essence beyond my being a thinking thing, I rightly conclude that my essence consists only in my being a thinking thing or a substance whose whole essence or nature is merely thinking. And although I may, or rather, as I will shortly say, although I certainly do possess a body with which I am very closely conjoined; nevertheless, because, on the one hand, I have a clear and distinct idea of myself, in as far as I am only a thinking and unextended thing, and as, on the other hand, I possess a distinct idea of body, in as far as it is only an extended and unthinking thing, *it is certain that I, that is, my mind, by which I am what I am, is entirely and truly distinct from my body, and may exist without it.* (emphasis added)

Both Descartes and Armstrong, therefore, consider that the only aspect of our mind that can truly be conceived as disembodied is mere self-awareness, that is, the consciousness of oneself as existing or being present. These quotes already contribute toward my thesis to the effect that the more mind you want to disembody, the more body you have to add to it, and, conversely, the less bodylike features you want to end up with in your conceived disembodiment scenario, the less realistic, or dumber mind you will have to conceive of. However, I want to also put forward three arguments of my own for this claim, based on three examples of experiences, increasing in complexity.

First, consider a simple experience of a brief sharp pain. Is it conceivable that this experience be disembodied in the relevant sense? Part of the phenomenology of such a state involves both a representation that the pain is located somewhere and the urge to act; for instance, if it is a burning sensation, it will be felt as being present or having happened somewhere in the body, and it will involve a reflex to remove that part of the body from the noxious source. Even if short, such a pain state is complex enough to conceptually involve the body. When you are in pain, something hurts; and it can't be that your mind as such hurts. It hurts somewhere in the body. So a state like this must involve a bodylike part at least, depending on how the pain phenomenally presents itself. It can be a body part like our actual body parts, or it can be a ghostly body part, or angelic, or psychic body part—it does not matter. What matters is that when you feel pain somewhere, you feel yourself as such hurt in that place, so you must have that place as a part of yourself. In other words, phenomenally, you feel yourself present in some located part of yours, feeling the urge to move yourself out of the way of whatever hurts you at that location. It is not as if you are totally unlocated and the pain that you feel is felt as merely *caused* at some location which does not contain you, a location that is alien to you. I call this argument "the argument from phenomenal location," its conclusion being that even the phenomenologically simplest and shortest experiential state does conceptually involve location of a body part.[16]

The second example involves a somewhat more complex and temporally more extended process, namely, chewing. Mastication, in normal subjects, takes place in an orderly way, in that its force depends on the felt texture and the hardness of the food. This is accounted for by a proprioceptive mechanism with peripheral components at the level of the teeth rather than the jaws (Schindler et al. 1998), so that the feedback from these has the role of guiding the chewing action of the jaws in such a way that it does not become injurious to the teeth. The force of the chewing is therefore exactly the right level for the food to be properly ground and the teeth not to get hurt. This reflex feedback mechanism is available to consciousness as such and available to attention in the dispositional sense. You

---

[16]An anonymous referee asks: Why can't the locations be *mere* appearances, that is, locations that aren't the real locations? Whether they are the real locations or not is not relevant here; what is relevant is that they must be thought of as *bodily* locations of some sort.

are aware that when you eat mashed potato, you do not really chew it at all, or that when you eat some lettuce salad and there is a little stone that failed to get eliminated when you washed the lettuce leaf, once your teeth come into contact with the hard stone, you stop chewing your salad and start exploring the contents of your mouth for a hard object; you chew much more carefully and try to single out the stone. How is the phenomenology of such chewing reflexes to be conceived as disembodied? It seems that beyond what we needed to posit in my previous example, which in the current example means the need to posit an oral cavity where the chewed food is felt as present, we also need to posit a mechanism that lies beyond the personal, subjective self because otherwise it would be impossible to explain the regularity of the phenomenal jaw movements as correlated with felt food textures and hardness. Why would an experience of chewing forcefully be followed by an experience of chewing carefully, when intercalated by the experience of a hard object in the mouthlike place? Such regularities require conceiving of a nonpersonal mechanism, which is itself at the level of a bodylike entity, be it biological body or ghostly quasi-body. Consequently, I call this argument "the argument from nonpersonal mechanisms." As a matter of fact, Descartes was well aware of such cases, but proposed, quite unconvincingly, that there might be a hidden mechanism which is still personal; that is, it has to do with the self as an essentially thinking thing. Here are two quotes supporting my claim:

> And although the perceptions of the senses were not dependent on my will, I did not think that I ought on that ground to conclude that they proceeded from things different from myself, since perhaps there might be found in me some faculty, though hitherto unknown to me, which produced them. (*Meditation* 6, part 7)
>
> Further, I cannot doubt but that there is in me a certain passive faculty of perception, that is, of receiving and taking knowledge of the ideas of sensible things; but this would be useless to me, if there did not also exist in me, or in some other thing, another active faculty capable of forming and producing those ideas. But this active faculty cannot be in me in as far as I am but a thinking thing, seeing that it does not presuppose thought, and also that those ideas are frequently produced in my mind without my contributing to it in any way, and even frequently contrary to my will. This faculty must therefore exist in some substance different from me, in which all the objective reality of the ideas that are produced by this faculty is contained formally or eminently, as I before remarked; and this substance is either a body, that is to say, a corporeal nature in which is contained formally and in effect all that is

objectively and by representation in those ideas; or it is God himself, or some other creature, of a rank superior to body, in which the same is contained eminently. *Meditation* 6, part 10

Setting aside the seeming contradiction between the two quotes (the first claiming that the perception producing mechanism is internal to oneself, but unknown yet, the second claiming that it must be based outside oneself, either in another body or God himself), Descartes is at pains trying to account for mental states that follow a regularity which is not up to the voluntary control of the thinking subject. He is compelled to admit the existence of a *mechanism*. First he states that the mechanism could be in the thinking subject itself, albeit in some yet unknown or obscure way, but later he admits that it must be taken as corporeal, quasi-corporeal, or divine.

Finally, consider an even more complex phenomenal state, the so-called Pinocchio illusion. It is a proprioceptive illusion that can be generated by applying a vibratory stimulus to the biceps joint. The subject is supposed to hold her nose with the arm whose biceps receives the vibration. The vibration excites the proprioceptive receptors in the muscle spindles and generates the illusory feeling that one's arm is extending. Since the hand of that arm is meantime touching the nose, subjects report that they feel their nose as growing, hence the name of the illusion. The belief that their nose is growing is, if we are to take their reports at face value, directly phenomenally based; they *feel* their own nose as growing. If we focused on all components of this complex state except the feeling of one's nose growing and we were a Cartesian disembodied mind, then we would form the same belief, but this time by logical inference. From "my arm is extending" and "I am touching my own nose with the hand of my extending arm" it follows (given some obvious assumptions) that my nose is growing. Yet, in actual fact we have the belief that our nose is growing directly, that is, non-inferentially. Consequently, we could call this argument "the argument from non-inferentiality." Again, this non-inferentiality of the belief requires us to posit a mechanism beyond the self as merely a thinking thing, and that mechanism will have to be thought of as involving bodylike structures.

To conclude, then, I agree that disembodiment is logically possible, however, in all such possibilities the mind that gets disembodied is very far from any realistic minds that people have around here in the actual world. Conversely, in all possibilities where a realistic mind is conceived, a bodylike, quasi-corporeal structure will inevitably be present too.

8

Against Action as
Constitutive of Mind

At the end of chapter 7, I mentioned the case of counting on one's fingers, advertised by Chalmers and Clark as a case of extended mind in their sense, which I claimed to be a case of embodied cognition. It is now time to substantiate this claim. In the first section of this chapter, I consider the case of counting on one's fingers as a potential case for embodied central processing. I argue that some aspects of it do qualify so, and hence the case qualifies as one of extended mind, although not one in which the mind extends beyond the nervous system. Second, in light of the discussion in the previous two chapters, I offer a brief critical review of some prominent embodied cognition theories that have been proposed recently, all of which award action a constitutive role to mind and especially to perception. I will argue that action itself, given the way I understand and define it, plays an important role in mental states, but it is most likely a causal rather than a constitutive role. The extant views are sensorimotor theories, whereas my own view about the embodied mind, as explained in the previous chapter, is a somatosensory theory. The difference is that while the former take both peripheral sensory input and action as constitutive of mental states, I only take peripheral sensory input as so.

I. *Embodied Central Processing*

Counting on one's fingers, or using one's fingers in order to perform a computation, is one of the plainest and most frequent cases of helping our central cognitive machinery work better by offloading some of its tasks onto a medium that lies outside the CNS. What exactly is involved in such a process? Is it a case of the finger movements constituting a central computational process, or is it one in which those movements are merely causally contributing to central processes? Earlier, in my discussion of Chalmers and Clark's extended mind hypothesis, I argued that the Tetris case is not one of extended central processing because there is peripheral mediation at the phenomenal level, that is, the phenomenology of pushing the buttons on a keyboard in order to rotate an image on the computer screen is such that it cannot count as the phenomenology associated with central processing. Now, this might be seen as being in tension with my claims in the first and the seventh chapter to the effect that the PNS is not felt as distinct from the self, but rather as a region where the self or mind extends and is entirely present. But there is no real tension here.

What I asserted regarding the Tetris case was that there is peripheral mediation between the subject, on the one hand, and the action applied to the button, as well as the way the figure on the screen appears, on the other hand. There is first a tactile peripheral mediation, which occurs between the subject and the surface of the buttons that are pushed on the keyboard in order to move the figures on the screen. And, second, there is visual peripheral mediation between the subject and the appearance of the figures on the computer screen. This mediation accounts, phenomenologically, for the process of rotating the figures as not being a central process proper, for the reasons I have put forward in chapter 6. But, of course, this is not to say that there is such a felt peripheral mediation between self and the motion of the fingers themselves when they hit the button, or between the self and the eyes that are focused on the screen. The eyes as such are not especially felt in any way as far as their visual function is concerned (though they are proprioceptively felt when, for instance, the large muscles that move the eyeball are used), whereas the fingers are felt as just part of oneself.

So what is the difference between pushing the button on the keyboard in order to change the appearance of the figure on the screen and the case of counting on one's fingers? The former case is one in which the two components, the keyboard and the screen, although used for the same purpose as a central process would use mental images, are felt as alien to oneself. The latter is one in which some peripheral nervous components, the moved fingers, are both used for the same purpose that a mental calculation would use memory and are felt as simply part of oneself. The calculation takes place as a matter of the interaction between higher cognitive and peripheral processes.

Yet, we have to distinguish several peripheral components of this complex process of counting on one's fingers, not all of which will turn out to be constitutively playing the role in what appears as central processing. Access to some of the peripheral components of this process are as much peripherally mediated, phenomenologically, as the access to the buttons and to the screen was in the Tetris case. For instance, some people's way of counting on their fingers involves a last stage of visual access to the fingers, just before the final solution to the computation is arrived at. This visual access to how many bent and how many straight fingers there are on one's hand is no different from the visual access one has to the computer screen in the Tetris case. Visually, the fingers are as alien to the self as any other external object.[1]

There is also a proprioceptively based, but, if I was right in the previous chapter, ultimately introspective component to the access to the state of one's fingers when counting. This occurs when people do not look at the fingers in order to ascertain their position (bent or straight) and their corresponding numbers, but merely focus on their muscular, skin stretch, and joint receptors, and learn these facts. If I was right in the previous chapter, when people do this, they, in fact, introspect rather than proprioceive proper. They focus their attention on what *they* feel regarding their hand and fingers, muscular tension, joint, and skin stretch. This process is far from being automatic, so if proprioception is a silent sense, this process is not to be counted as proprioceptive but introspective. The contents of what is presented to the introspecting subject in this case bring about almost as much phenomenologically peripheral mediation between the fingers and the self as the Tetris case did between the screen and the self, or the visual access did when the fingers were visually attended to. I say "almost as much phenomenologically peripheral

[1] This is why deafferented subjects, that is, subjects who suffered complete loss of sensory nerves below the neck, even though they can adapt to their new condition and live a normal life via replacing proprioceptive information with visual information, should not be considered as really counting on their fingers when they visually control and acknowledge their fingers' position in order to calculate. The way normal subjects count on their fingers is essentially proprioceptive, whereas the deafferented subjects' use of the fingers is exclusively visual, hence it is inessential whether the subject used her fingers or any other externally available physical support. But, as I explain below, counting on one's fingers is far from using the fingers as one among many possible external devices; they are in fact not external at all. For more information about a case of deafferented human subject, see Gallagher and Cole 1995.

mediation" because, on the one hand, the fingers in this case certainly do not feel as alien, yet, on the other hand, they are treated as part of an introspectively formed and accessed image, unlike when they are used for various motor tasks, in which case they enter consciousness more directly, and in fact constitutively, if the main philosophical hypothesis of this book is right, even though more silently than when focusing one's attention on them.

Finally, there is a peripheral component to the process of counting on one's fingers which is truly proprioceptive, and hence access to the fingers in this case is not phenomenologically peripherally mediated, so it counts as a constitutive part of the central process of computing.

Now, when Clark and Chalmers say that "counting on our fingers has already been let in the door, for example, and it is easy to push things further" (1998: 11), we need to only be clear about *which* aspect or component of counting on one's fingers, of the ones mentioned above, has really been let in the door. The relevant component is the purely proprioceptive one, which is phenomenologically peripherally unmediated, hence can qualify as computing. This component is located in the PNS, so its involvement in computing extends, indeed, the process beyond the CNS, but it is not extra-neural altogether. Therefore, the counting on fingers is extended, but not beyond the nervous system; it is a case of embodied cognition rather than extended mind in Chalmers and Clark's sense.

II. *The Conceptual Role of the Neuromuscular Junction*

Philosophers of mind use a lot terms like "motor action" or "behavior," in the context of trying to offer a picture of mentality, a context in which the referent of these terms is going to be integrated in a functional description of the mental states in question. Yet, not many of them have found it worth trying to analyze these terms.[2] From a neurophysiological point of view, philosophers who championed a functional description and analysis of mental states have always implicitly assumed that behavior or motor action is a type of neural event that occurs immediately after the CNS has done its job on a stimulus, that is, a type of PNS event. As according to our hypothesis mental states are extended through the nervous system

----

[2] An exception is Ruth Millikan (1993: ch. 7), but her focus is biology, whereas I focus here on neurophysiology.

in its entirety, behavior proper is going to refer to events in the body that are *extra-neural*, events that occur past the *neuromuscular junction*, in the typical cases of behavior. The typical such event is muscle contraction in any part of the body. The neuromuscular junction is then, both conceptually and empirically, the mind-behavior boundary. As any boundary, its own status will not allow us to classify it under either "mental state" or "behavior," but that is not a problem. There are many other such theoretical boundaries in neuroscience that we are not supposed to determinately classify in one of the categories that it distinguishes. The best example is the distinction between the CNS and the PNS. Although we assume the distinction is unproblematic, there is a region in the spinal cord where most afferent peripheral nerve fibers enter deeply and connect to the neurons of the spine, called "the transitional region" (TR), so that strictly speaking this region is neither exclusively part of the CNS, nor that of the PNS, as it contains tissue belonging to both:

> the TR is the most proximal free part of the root which in one and the same cross-section contains both CNS and PNS tissue. The term transitional region has been chosen rather than "entry zone," "junction," or "border" because it gives greater emphasis to the conceptual importance of the structural changes that take place in association with a more extended and spacious structure than is indicated by the other terms.... The interface between the axial CNS compartment and the surrounding PNS compartment is referred to as the CNS–PNS borderline, which is penetrated by nerve fibers. In this way, nerve fibers in the PNS extend into the CNS or vice versa and thus traverse the TR. This region therefore holds a position of conceptual importance with regard to neuronal organization as well as a model system for experimental investigations regarding differences in reaction patterns within one and the same neuron in the two main parts of the nervous system. (Carlstedt et al. 2004: 251, 253)

Like the TR, the neuromuscular junction (NMJ) should also hold a position of conceptual importance, namely, when it comes to a precise understanding of the notion of action or behavior. The NMJ is the location at which the neuron activates the muscle causing it to contract. Neurologically, it is the last synapse that takes place before the relevant muscle contracts. Anatomically, it is the place where the motor neuron acts upon the muscular end plate, the highly excitable muscle fiber membrane responsible for transmitting the action potentials to groups of muscle fibers. The substance that exclusively realizes the synapse at the NMJ in motor action of the

S*omatic Nervous System* (e.g., voluntary muscle action) is the neurotransmitter *acetylcholine* (ACh), whereas in the *Autonomic Nervous System* (e.g., heart rate, sweating, and other such reflexes) we find several such neurotransmitters, beside ACh.

Now, philosophers of mind have been talking about a functional analysis of mental states, again, in a way that neglects important neuroscientific details. The philosophers' preferred way of explaining the functionalist understanding of a mental state is by saying something like: "a mental state M can be analyzed as the state caused by such-and-such stimuli and causing, together with other mental states, such-and-such behavior." Then typically they add that details don't matter, as this is a purely conceptual matter. I agree that we might take the feasibility of such an analysis as a purely conceptual matter, but I don't see why it should follow that details do not matter. There are scientific conceptual details, beyond the above-mention superficial exposition of functionalism, that *do* matter. One such detail is the question of what to say about behavior when it comes to placing it relative to the NMJ. Although I could not find any philosopher who thought about this issue, I think most of them implicitly think of behavior as whatever occurs in the motor neurons, that is, just outside the CNS in the efferent component of the PNS.

According to my hypothesis and the corresponding *total state functionalism* (where a mental state involves both the CNS and the PNS), a mental state will be the causal link between a stimulus, understood as an extra-neural event, and behavior, understood as an event occurring past the NMJ, so extra-neural. This way of characterizing mental states, stimuli, and behavior is at least as adequate empirically as the orthodox way, which circumscribes mental states by appeal to the boundaries of the brain or the CNS. Moreover, a good case can be made for the view based on some examples when it is more intuitive to think of behavior in the way I have circumscribed it, namely, as occurring past the NMJ.

Take first the case of general anesthesia effected on some subjects who are about to undergo surgery. It is usual that general anesthesia consists of administering two drug components: an anesthetic or analgesic drug and a muscle relaxant. Sometimes the muscle relaxant is a neuromuscular blocker, which means that the drug acts at the NMJ, by inhibiting ACh synthesis or release. What is the reason for administering the neuromuscular blocker? It is to make sure that the patient's muscular activity is reduced to zero, so that the possibility of motor activity that might interfere with the correct surgical procedure is eliminated. In other words, what the surgeon wants is to eliminate *behavior* on the part of the patient during the operation. This is needed because, regardless of how strong the general anesthetic which renders the CNS unconscious is, it is an empirical fact that behavior can still occur. Since the blocking takes place at the NMJ, we can deduce that there still is in many cases of rendering the CNS unconscious neural activity at the level of the efferent (motor) peripheral nerve fibers. Yet, the action of the neuromuscular blocker counts as behavior-blocking. Intuitively, we would not say of a patient who is paralyzed by neuromuscular blocking agents that she still behaves in some way, perhaps to a lesser extent. We simply say that behavior is rendered impossible by rendering the NMJ inactive. What follows is that the essence of behavior is not the activity of the motor part of the PNS, but the activity of the tissues that are innervated by those motor nerve fibers.[3] In other words, the activity of the motor part of the PNS is not sufficient for the concept of behavior to apply, although it is necessary, since the function of the NMJ involves transmission of the nervous signal to the muscular end plate.

As a second example, consider the case of neurological investigations including nerve conduction and reaction time studies. What these studies aim to ultimately establish is the time between the activation of a stimulus and the onset of the relevant muscular action. It is ultimately behavior considered as muscular action that is of interest rather than the activation of the motor part of the PNS per se.

This discussion will be relevant at the end of the following section, where I try to formulate a rough theory of the place action should have in a theory of mind, and more precisely of perception.

III. A Brief Critique of Action-Based (Sensorimotor) Theories

The new, embodied approach to philosophy of mind and cognitive science is usually contrasted by its proponents with classical or orthodox cognitive science and sometimes with what some authors label as "Cartesian cognitive science" (e.g., Rowlands 2010). I myself

---

[3] Of course, not all muscle relaxants act at the level of the NMJ; a second category is that of drugs acting centrally, known as *spasmolytic* drugs. In that case the blocking takes place before the NMJ, at the level of the CNS. However, my point is that since the neuromuscular blockers do count as behavior-blockers, blocking the muscle is indeed essential to blocking behavior, hence, by contraposition, muscular activity is essential to the concept of behavior.

asserted earlier in this book that I find sympathy in the anti-Cartesian approach of the embodied mind movement, although, to be fair, there is a lot of textual evidence that Descartes himself was not very Cartesian in the sense in which this term is used today in cognitive science. For instance, the passages I quoted from Descartes in the previous chapter show a much more complex picture than the parody of Descartes that we usually find in contemporary nonhistorical philosophy of mind and cognitive science. However, this book is not the right place to elaborate on a defense of Descartes, so I will adopt the label "Cartesian" for the sake of differentiating the embodied approach from and contrasting it with the orthodox cognitive science, just like proponents of this approach themselves do.

Various authors attribute various features to orthodox cognitive science, but there are two features that most embodied mind theorists mention. One is internalism in the form of what Putnam called "methodological solipsism," and the other is the view that cognition is a rule-based process of manipulating symbolic representations.[4] Let us briefly explain these ideas. Internalism or methodological solipsism has already been explained in our chapter 5, where I discussed the issue of whether the bounds of the mind are extra-neural, that is, constitutively dependent upon facts outside the body. Methodological solipsism is the doctrine that mental states are based on representations which are, as a matter of principle, independent of an external world; in the extreme, even if the external world ceased to exist mental states could still survive. In other words, mental states are to be understood as self-sufficient, as states whose content is not necessarily affected by changes or states of affairs in the world and even in the body.

The second feature implies that representations are to be understood as some more or less complex symbols that undergo processing in the CNS and especially in the higher cortical areas, so that at the end of the process the conscious mental state emerges. Marr's theory of vision, which we briefly discussed in chapter 2, is an example of the classic approach.

The embodied approach has by now a respectable history, starting from the 1980s, where one can identify several stages. I do not intend in this book to review this history and to expound in detail whatever has been proposed in the literature, as it has been done by several authors, some of whom were involved in the development of this approach. I will rather briefly criticize the newest and most

[4] Cf. Menary 2007 and Rowlands 2010.

successful development in this area, namely, *Enactivism.* However, a brief presentation of the main different strands and the guiding ideas is worth presenting here.

There are roughly two stages and several types of approach that can be considered as self-proclaimed new cognitive science, in opposition to classical computationalism. The emergence of connectionism can be considered a kind of postclassical stage, whereas the embodied and embedded mind approach (EE) can be considered as anticlassical. Connectionism emerged as an alternative to classicism's view of the mind as a computer that processes symbolic language. The picture offered by connectionism is that of neural networks, whose connectivity properties explain learning and skill acquisition by the cognitive system. Classicism is a top-down approach, where complex symbols are fundamental and irreducible, whereas the neural networks picture is a bottom-up approach, where the activity of the networks generates and explains relevant mental phenomena. The advantage of connectionism is in that it appears as empirically more adequate when it comes to perception and sensation, as well as learning based on experience.[5] However, as far as connectionism goes, cognition could still work or be understood as a disembodied process, where what matters is what happens inside a neural network that is governed by internal or endogenous rules and states. Indeed, one of the proponents of the dynamic systems approach to cognition, which I take as part of a second stage, that of anticlassical cognitive science, has criticized connectionism along these lines pointing out that the main difference between classicism and connectionism is that the former conceives of computation as serial whereas the latter is based on the idea of parallel and distributed computation, but that is not a difference from the point of view of whether methodological solipsism is questioned or excluded from one's theory (e.g., Beer, forthcoming). The dynamic systems approach is based on the mathematical theory of dynamic systems, which defines and analyzes the evolution of various abstract dynamic systems. A dynamic system consists of a number of initial condition states that the system can be in, a rule for the evolution of the system, a state space consisting of all the possible states that the systems can be in, and equilibria (steady states or attractors) of the system which generate stability (i.e., no further change) of the system. Theorists involved in the dynamic systems approach tend to

---

[5] For detailed accounts, see Rumelhart, McClelland, and the PDP Research Group 1986, Smolensky 1988, and Bechtel and Abrahamsen 1991.

emphasize their commitment to an interaction among brain, body, and environment as fundamental to any dynamic understanding of cognition.[6]

The dynamic system approach is part of the EE approach. Another strand in the EE approach, besides the Extended Mind hypothesis, which I discussed in chapter 6 and in the first section of this chapter, is *Enactivism*, which seems to be today the most popular view that claims to offer something beyond and in opposition to classical cognitive science. The approach is taken to originate in Varela, Thompson, and Rosch's 1991 book, *The Embodied Mind: Cognitive Science and Human Experience*, where the basis of most of the discussion that followed was laid. The book is interdisciplinary and quite eclectic, combining analytic philosophy of mind, Continental philosophy, Husserl's and Merleau-Ponty's phenomenology, Buddhism, and cognitive science. While several ideas, such as the Buddhist component, have not succeeded in making much of a career during the years that followed, some other ideas, most notably the idea that action is essential to perception would subsequently galvanize discussion on the subject and be responsible for the emergence of the latest monographs published under the heading of embodied mind. This current popularity of enactivism is the reason I would like to discuss it and offer a critical view to contrast it with my own version of the embodied mind, namely, the PMH.

One idea that is common to enactive approaches—and is currently subscribed to by a growing number of philosophers of mind—is that action plays an essential role in perception. As it stands, this point is not clear enough. Let us start with a quote from Varela, Thompson, and Rosch (VTR):

> We can now give a preliminary formulation of what we mean by *enaction*. In a nutshell, the enactive approach consists of two points: (1) perception consists in perceptually guided action and (2) cognitive structures emerge from the recurrent sensorimotor patterns that enable action to be perceptually guided. (1991: 173)

What VTR mean when they say that perception consists in perceptually guided action is that the organism is not a passive receiver of stimulation from the environment, but it creates its own stimulation situations via action. In the end, we should not analyze perception according to a "snapshot conception," but rather as the dynamic

---

[6] For the dynamic systems approach, see Thelen and Smith 1994, Beer 2000, and Van Gelder 1995, 1998.

structure of action guidance, where the ultimate unit of analysis is holistic, consisting of cycles of perception–action–perception– .... As VTR themselves point out, Merleau-Ponty made this point earlier, for instance, in the following passage:

> The organism cannot properly be compared to a keyboard on which the external stimuli would play and in which their proper form would be delineated for the simple reason that the organism contributes to the constitution of that form.... When the eye and the ear follow an animal in flight, it is impossible to say "which started first" in the exchange of stimuli and responses. Since all the movements of the organism are always conditioned by external influences, one can, if one wishes, readily treat behavior as an effect of the milieu. But in the same way, since all the stimulations which the organism receives have in turn been possible only by its preceding movements which have culminated in exposing the receptor organ to external influences, one could also say that *behavior is the first cause of all the stimulations.* (quoted in Varela, Thompson, and Rosch 1991: 173–74) (emphasis in original)

Now we can ask the following question: What is so special about the idea that action, or self-initiated movement is involved in a series consisting of successive perceptual experiences that it should count as something radically different from so-called "classical cognitive science"? The reply must be that action or behavior should be taken as constitutive of the elements in that series of perceptual experiences. But, for all we learn from either VTR or Merleau-Ponty, action is simply a cause of perception. Merleau-Ponty emphatically adds that behavior is "the first cause of all the stimulation," but it is hard to see in what sense it is a first cause, since a cause is just an event among a long series of past and future causes and effects. If he means that it is a constitutive element of perception, then this much does not follow from the fact that it causally acts on the relevant set of stimuli. There is not yet any argument, for instance, of the kind I have offered in the previous chapter as to why we should consider action as constitutive of perception.[7]

Alva Noë (2004) seems to offer a more elaborate view on this matter, so maybe his theory of perception as sensorimotor knowledge

---

[7] And there is an even more fundamental problem, as noted by Schellenberg (2010: 155), namely, that for all we are told, it is not necessary that the change in the stimulation originates in the motor action of the perceiving subject; it could be generated by some other (natural or artificial) agent moving the objects themselves for the perceiving agent, or even the agents body parts being moved by such an external device, say, via remote control. Mere movement is not the same thing as action, so if all that is needed for perception is past and counterfactual experience of motion, then this view does not amount to claiming that action is constitutive of perception.

will fare better in terms of convincing us that action must be taken as constitutive of perception. According to this view, to perceive an object involves at least past knowledge and counterfactual knowledge of how one could act on or relative to that object. To perceive a bottle by touch involves not simply touching it, but having some implicit knowledge of how it could be further touched on different regions of it and how it, or something similar, was touched in the past. To visually perceive a backpack involves not simple presentation in view of the backpack, but knowledge of so-called practical conditionals about how the object would appear from different angles and/or how it, or something similar, used to appear from different angles, how one would move or has moved around the object, and so on. This sensorimotor knowledge, then, constitutes the perception in situ of any object in one's environment, so that perception is not to be understood on a snapshot view according to which it merely involves the stimulation of the senses from the environment and the neural processing of that raw information.

The way Noë puts his thesis several times in his book is that in order to perceive we need "knowledge of sensorimotor contingencies." This sounds implausible, mainly because *knowledge* of such sensorimotor contingencies (e.g., practical counterfactuals of the form "if I moved to the left, I would experience the object as such-and-such") is a higher cognitive state, which one would expect to be a constitutive part of at most perceptual *judgment*, not of perception as such. In other words, prima facie, the sensorimotor theory is not a theory of what and how we perceive, but of how we think or conceptualize what we perceive. A second problem, noted by Jesse Prinz (2006: 3), is that to use the expression "sensorimotor" in the account of perception, which obviously involves sensory states, is circular. You try to offer an account of sensation by appeal to knowledge of sensation, among other things.

However, both Noë and other authors who promote enactivism, appeal to knowledge as *skill*, which should be interpreted as implicit rather than explicit. Thus, Noë asserts that "to perceive you must be in possession of sensorimotor bodily skill" (2004: 11). Noë further asserts (chapter 6) that sensorimotor knowledge is subpersonal. Things become more complicated when he also claims that perception is a kind of understanding, a "thoughtful activity," and that it is partly conceptual. His motivation for these latter claims is that we should not think that whatever is conceptual and thoughtlike cannot be subpersonal, skill-like, and implicit. Let us grant all these points to Noë and focus rather on one of the main empirical bases that he considers for his view, the case of inverting goggles.

In one such experiment, subjects are asked to wear goggles that invert the left-right orientation in space, so that the new experience of the environment should intuitively represent objects that are truly on the right as being on the left and vice versa. In another, they are asked to wear goggles that invert the up-down spatial axis, so that objects should appear upside down. As the philosophers' story goes, subjects at first have a truly chaotic, destructured experience of their environment, after which they see the world as inverted according as what kind of inverting goggles they wear, and, finally and more importantly, after a while their experience adapts to the world, or it "veridicalizes" itself, to use Noë's way of putting it, so that they experience the environment as it really is. The reason why the experience veridicalizes itself is because the subjects are involved, during the training for wearing the glasses, in various motor activities, so that ultimately it is because of these activities that experience adapts to the new condition, given that the sensory stimulation of the retina stays constant (as long as the glasses are on). Both Noë and Susan Hurley (1998: ch. 9) are convinced that the results of these experiments are evidence that supports their sensorimotor view. What enactivists take as "the result" of such experiments is that perception after wearing inverting goggles "reinverts" itself so as to correspond to the objective facts in the environment. Unfortunately, none of the experiments are described in proper detail in any of the books of the enactivists, which leaves out important details that make a difference when it comes to evaluating their theory with respect to experimental evidence. I am not the first one to point out that, as a matter of fact, this supposed result of reinversion of the experience has not been established; Colin Klein (2007) has done it before. On the contrary, more recent studies show evidence against this claim. Klein quotes a study by Linden et al. 1999:

> Subjects, who wore prism- and mirror-inverting spectacles over periods of six to ten days, showed a rapid visuomotor adaptation and were able to interact correctly with the surrounding world after a few days. This adaptation was not accompanied by a return of upright vision, as assessed by introspection, reading performance, and the extraction of three-dimensional shape from shading.... This dissociation of visuomotor and perceptual adaptation contradicts established views about the changes brought about by inversions of visual input. (2007: 612)

Moreover, Klein is right in pointing out that neither Stratton (1897) nor Kohler (1961, [1951] 1964), the two pioneering studies that both

Noë and Hurley partly rely on to argue for enactivism, have taken their experiments to have shown that perception "veridicalizes" after exposure of the eyes to inverting goggles:

> Kohler writes that Dr. von Kundratitz was biking by the fourth day of the experiment and skiing by the sixth, yet, "During all this time, however, his perceptions were only sporadically rightside up." Similarly, "During a simulated fencing match, the subject parried all blows correctly, even though the opponent was seen upside-down." (Klein 2007: 613)

So *the subjects' own testimony*, that is, their first-person reports, actually contradict what Noë would like to see in these experiments. However, I want to focus on a different detail, which has evaded even Klein's and other critics' attention. There is a certain irresoluteness across various writings by Noë and Hurley about what to say and in how to interpret what happens when the goggles are *removed*. Here are three quotes, each of which emphasizes something different about this case, so that the data seems overall contradictory, and yet, the authors always use it to support their sensorimotor hypothesis.

The first quote is from Noë (2004: 9–10), where in connection to Kohler's 1964 findings he says:

> Once full adaptation has been achieved, the result in *removing* the lenses is comparable to the initial effects of putting them on. Taking the lenses off induces exactly the same kind of experiential blindness, and for exactly the same reasons that putting them on did at first: The glasses (or their absence) cause a sudden abrogation of the patterns of dependence of sensation and movement.

Noë takes this to clearly support the sensorimotor theory in that it shows that "perceptual experience acquires content as a result of sensorimotor knowledge" (2004: 9).

But then we find another quote, this time from Hurley and Noë (2003: 163), where, in connection with work by James Taylor (1963) involving inverting goggles, they report that there are cases when such a disruption of visual experience when removing the glasses— "experiential blindness" to use Noë's own (and in my opinion quite misleading) expression—does not occur, but Noë and Hurley do not seem to be bothered by such cases; on the contrary, they think these cases also support their sensorimotor knowledge hypothesis:

> Taylor reports that one of his long-term subjects experienced no aftereffect when removing or reinstating the goggles (while riding a bicycle!). This suggests a very striking variability in qualitative expression. With goggles on, left arm stimulates RV-cortex, and looks leftward. With

goggles off, right arm stimulates RV-cortex, and looks rightward. Here, the qualitative expression of activity in RV-cortex would vary between 'looks rightward' and 'looks leftward'. The subject has acquired know-how in relation to both sets of patterns of sensorimotor contingencies, with and without goggles, and switches between them seamlessly.

It looks like whatever happens when the glasses are removed, disruption or no change at all, Noë and/or Hurley seem to think that it supports their view. On the condition that what happens when glasses are removed is relevant, this simply cannot be right.

Finally, here is a third quote, this time from Taylor, which Hurley uses to emphasize the lack of any disturbance when the glasses are removed:

> As predicted, adaptation was not blocked by the daily periods of normal vision. On the contrary, it was more rapid than it had been in the two previous experiments in Innsbruck, and this can doubtless be attributed to the systematic training described above. Also, there was no disruption of behavior when the spectacles were put on or taken off. And finally, the prediction that the right-left ordering of the perceptual field would remain unchanged when the spectacles were put on or removed was confirmed. This was strikingly illustrated when the subject rode a bicycle while wearing the spectacles, and took them off and replaced them without changing course or wobbling or showing any other sign of disruption. Objects that he perceived as being on his left while wearing the spectacles were still on his left when he took them off. (Taylor 1963: 204, quoted by Hurley 1998: 349)

Again, it is hard to see how to corroborate all these observations and emphases into a coherent whole meant to support enactivism, given that they are contradictory. The issue of whether visual perceptual changes occur at all when subjects adapt to wearing the experimental spectacles is controversial in the psychological literature itself; it is not a philosopher's puzzle exclusively. Harris (1963, 1965), for instance, has argued, based on an extensive review of the literature and on his own experiments, that there is no *visual* change after adaptation in the sense of pictorial representation, and that adaptation is grounded in proprioceptive changes.[8] However, I would like to return to the studies of Benedetti on subjects with crossed fingers because one of Benedetti's goals was to gain new insights from other

---

[8] Noë and Hurley (2003) and Noë (2004) do provide extensive criticism of Harris 1965.

sense modalities that could tell something about the more discussed visual case. As we will see, the results explain, by analogy, the apparent contradictoriness in data about what happens when the goggles are taken off, and they do not support enactivism; moreover, I will argue that they actually disprove enactivism.

The effects of taking the experimental spectacles off are called "aftereffects" in the literature, and as far as vision is concerned it is seldom made clear what aftereffects occur when, namely, after how much training, that is, wearing the glasses. This is the culprit in the apparent incoherence of the three quotes above. The strong aftereffects (disruption of the visual field) that Noë finds relevant to emphasize in the first quote are, if we extrapolate the tactile study I am going to describe to vision, phenomena that occur early in the training period, whereas in later stages adaptation in both the normal and inverted conditions will have occurred, with apparently seamless, nondisruptive transition between the two states.

The study by Benedetti that I have discussed (Benedetti 1991) is relevant here. His goal was to test what happens in terms of perceptual learning after long-lasting tactile reversal. Perceptual learning itself has been divided into two components: perceptual performance and motor performance. Tactile reversal at the level of the fingers is easier to bring about than visual reversal, as you do not need a special device, like the experimental goggles in the case of vision. All you need is to keep a pair of fingers crossed for a certain time. The subjects have their fingers crossed during the day and uncrossed during sleep, but even during the day they could uncross them any time they wanted. A total of six subjects participated in the experiment, the shortest period of experimental conditions (i.e., fingers crossed) being 60 days, the longest being 121 days. In addition to the daily tactile exploration of the environment, subjects underwent more intense training three times a week, with both crossed and uncrossed fingers, during which they explored objects under visual guidance. For example, one instance of such training was to explore a larger ball and a point, each touching one of the fingers, crossed and uncrossed.

One instance of how perceptual performance was tested was by applying the stimuli for a longer time, 3 s, and asking the subject to judge the position of the ball with respect to the point (e.g., to the left or to the right of the point). Motor performance, on the other hand, involved a shorter application of the tactile stimuli, 500 ms, and asking the subject to move the hand toward the target stimulus, for example, ball or point (e.g., the subject is briefly touched by the ball on one finger and point on the other, then asked to move his or her hand toward where the ball was felt as touching from). It is important that in both types of tests the stimuli were shielded from view and the subjects were not given feedback on whether their choices were correct.

The results were as follows. As opposed to an earlier study (Benedetti 1990), in which subjects were given feedback on their motor performance, and which demonstrated that motor performance with crossed fingers increases considerably *within the first hour* of training, when subjects are not given feedback, motor performance in the inverted condition increases much slower, reaching 100 percent accuracy in about two and a half months. The motor performance in the normal condition (uncrossed fingers) *decreases* for about a month, then it is stable for another month, then it increases for another two weeks, and reaches 100 percent accuracy at the same time as the motor performance in the inverted condition (i.e., two and a half months since the beginning of the experiment). These are the data on motor performance.

Perceptual performance stays constant at the initial level of accuracy in the normal condition for the whole period of the experiment. Perceptual performance in the inverted condition, on the other hand, increases in accuracy steadily, but slower than motor performance increases in that condition, namely, it reaches full accuracy in about six months (as opposed to motor performance in the inverted condition, whose accuracy reaches 100 percent in two and a half months). The results are synthesized in the graph in figure 8.1, where solid lines indicate motor and perceptual performance in

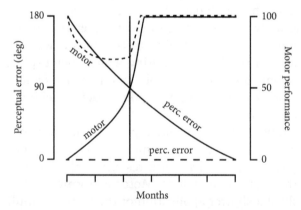

Figure 8.1 Perceptual error versus motor performance in tactile recognition tasks with crossed fingers. (Redrawn from Benedetti 1991)

the inverted condition, whereas dashed lines indicate those in the normal condition.

There are several observations to make that have an impact on the issue of whether enactivism is supported or not by experiments involving inversion. Focusing on the results of this study on tactile inversion, the first thing to notice is that behavior in the form of motor performance adapts to the new condition a lot earlier that perception does. As it is apparent on the graph, the time difference between complete motor performance adaptation to inversion and perceptual adaptation is no less than three months! The results that Noë is impressed by in the first quote, namely, that the effect of removing the glasses, "once full adaptation has been achieved," is disruptive is most likely an effect that occurs early in the training, and what Kohler refers to by using the phrase "full adaptation" is motor performance *in the condition of feedback on one's action*, which is almost unavoidable in the visual case.[9] We know from the earlier study by Benedetti (1990) that with such feedback subjects learn to perform correctly and this learning is entirely cognitive, not perceptual:

> In fact, in Benedetti (1990) I demonstrated that motor learning was exclusively cognitive during the first hour of training; that is, without any perceptual learning, what the subjects learned was to perform the movement opposite that required for target reaching. (Benedetti 1991: 275)

So it is likely that the quick adaptation (coupled with the disruptive aftereffects) that Noë mentions in the first quote, apparently in support of enactivism, is not perceptual yet, but exclusively cognitive. This would not be a problem if Noë's enactivism weren't based on sensorimotor knowledge, which, as he himself emphasizes, is cognitive and conceptual. The problem is that if this kind of enactivism were true, then perceptual learning and adaptation should occur roughly at the same time as motor learning, and the curves of their improvement should follow each other closely because the knowledge of sensorimotor contingencies very shortly after inversion is as good as it gets. But the time discrepancy between these two types of adaptation, behavioral and perceptual, is considerable, three months in the above experiment, so I conclude that Noë's enactivism is not supported by data.

---

[9] It is very hard to think of an experimental setup that would filter perceptual from motor performance in the case of visual inversion, although I don't exclude that it might be practically possible.

So what is the role of action or behavior as such in perception, if not a constitutive one as enactivism would have us accept? The points I made in the second section of this chapter regarding the concept of behavior are relevant here. It looks to me that action as such—that is, the events taking place past the NMJ—has an important role in that it potentially presents the perceiver with a series of newer and newer aspects of the objects that one is in contact with, but this role is merely causal, not conceptual or constitutive in some way. Part of my perceiving a small cube might be causally determined by my being able to act on it, manipulate it, and so on, but the mere acts of manipulation seem to only causally contribute to my representation of the object as a cube. However, besides the mere act of manipulating, one can identify the phenomenon of sensing that one is manipulating the object. My hypothesis is that to the extent that action-related phenomena constitutively enter perception, they will have to be sensory or rather *somatosensory*. The somatosensory system include tactile perception, sensing one's position and motion, as well as sensing one's own muscles.

Several authors, including the enactivists I have been discussing above, have pointed out, based on experimental results (Held 1961; Held and Bossom 1961; Held and Freedman 1963; Held and Rekosh 1963; Held and Hein 1963), that active movement plays a crucial role in adaptation to perceptual distortion. Experimental evidence suggests that such adaptation takes place much quicker when subjects are asked to actively explore their environment (e.g., by walking around and manipulating objects) than when they are exploring them passively (e.g., by being taken around on a wheelchair). Enactivists appeal to these facts in order to support their own view. Here is, for instance, a quote from Noë (2004: 13):

> Held and Hein (1963) performed an experiment in which two kittens were harnessed to a carousel. One of the kittens was harnessed in such a way that it stood firmly on the ground. The other kitten was suspended in the air. As the one kitten walked, both kitten moved in a circle. As a result, they received identical visual stimulation, but only one of them received that stimulation as a result of self-movement. Remarkably (but not surprisingly from an enactive point of view), only the self-moving kitten developed normal depth perception (not to mention normal paw-eye coordination). From an enactive standpoint, we can venture an explanation for this: Only through *self*-movement can one *test* and so *learn* the relevant patterns of sensorimotor knowledge.

However, it is far from obvious that these findings actually support enactivism. If sensorimotor knowledge is based, as enactivists make it clear, on practical counterfactuals of the form "if you effect movement M, you will have sensation S," so that the role movement plays is to expose various aspects of the environment to sensory access, then whether the subjects of perceptual distortion explore the environment actively or passively should not make a difference to perceptual learning, since the experimental setup for passive exploration can easily match that of active exploration in terms of the series of aspects of the environment that become available as experience unfolds. What the experiments show is that behavior is indeed important for perceptual adaptation, but *not* in virtue of making various aspects of the environment available as sensorimotor cycles unfold, but rather in virtue of its *somatosensory* component, that is, the proprioceptive and kinesthetic phenomena associated with action. If this is so, then it is not action that is constitutive to perception, for instance, to visual perception, but rather proprioception and kinesthesia. This is my somatosensory hypothesis regarding perception, and, in effect, this is how, for example, Harris (1965) interprets perceptual adaptation in the context of distorting prisms and goggles.

Part IV

Mind and Ethics

9

Issues in Neuroethics

Neuroethics is a nascent interdisciplinary field concerned with several topics, connected by the general claim that ethics and neuroscience could benefit from each other. There have been several potential definitions of neuroethics proposed by various authors in order to circumscribe its field, but a straightforward and intuitive way to understand it, due to Adina Roskies (2002), is to break it down to two components: the ethics of neuroscience and the neuroscience of ethics. The former deals with ethical issues that arise in connection with neuroscientific practice, such as experimentation, invasive and noninvasive neurocognitive intervention, psycho-pharmacotherapy, and neurocognitive rehabilitation. The latter deals with a potential naturalistic reduction of many classic ethical concepts and problems to neurocognitive facts. In a most general way to put it, neuroethics would be an interdisciplinary field dealing with ethics with a view on the nervous system and with neuroscience with a view on ethics.

One thing that strikes me when reading various programmatic pieces about neuroethics is that all authors, without exception, mention the brain as the only relevant anatomical unit when it comes to neuroethical issues and puzzles. Here are some examples.

In her programmatic article about neuroethics, Roskies asserts that:

> The intimate connection between our brains and our behaviors, as well as the peculiar relationship between our brains and our selves, generate distinctive questions that beg for the interplay between ethical and neuroscientific thinking.... Many of us overtly or covertly believe in a kind of "neuroessentialism," that our brains define who we are, even more than do our genes. So in investigating the brain, we investigate the self. (2002: 21)

Michael Gazzaniga, one of the pioneers of the field, titles his book *The Ethical Brain* and writes that neuroethics deals with:

> the social issues of disease, normality, mortality, lifestyle, and the philosophy of living, informed by our understanding of underlying brain mechanisms....It is—or should be—an effort to come up with a brain-based philosophy of life. (2005: xv)

Then Colin Blakemore adds:

> If one accepts that the brain, and the brain alone, is responsible for the entirety of consciousness and action, including the sense of right and wrong, and the capacity to contemplate moral values, then it is legitimate to ask whether there is any sort of ethics other than neuroethics. (2006: v)

Finally, Patricia Churchland notes:

> Philosophers and others are now struggling to understand the significance of seeing morality not as a product of supernatural processes, 'pure reason' or so called 'natural law', but of brains. (2006: 3)

Even without subscribing to our peripheral mind thesis one can easily question this brain-centeredness when it comes to neuroethical issues. Let's take a simple case. Suppose John has a chronic sodium imbalance at the level of his blood plasma, and hence at the level of all bodily tissues, with a lot more salt retention than normal. He is on the road and is very thirsty, so he stops to buy some water. He realizes he has lost his wallet and has only one dollar worth of change in some corner of his pocket. He buys a small bottle of water and drinks it, but his thirst is far from being quenched, so he steals a couple of bottles, after the seller refuses to offer him water for free. Now, legally, his chronic condition of plasma sodium imbalance will most probably be a mitigating factor in court, if he is accused of stealing. Does the brain state he was in when stealing, as compared to the biochemistry of his blood and organ tissues, have more importance and impact on such a judgment as to whether health-based mitigating factors existed when he committed the crime? Intuitively, no. On the contrary, judges would most probably not go as far as to check his brain states when in such a state of sodium imbalance. A simple blood test would do just as well.[1]

---

[1] An anonymous referee suggests that it is the subject's belief that is exculpatory, not the truth maker of that belief, so even if he, unbeknownst to him, got cured of his illness, he would still have some moral justification to steal the bottle. All I said

You might think this example works only because it is about a very "low-level" mental state, namely, thirst, and that the interesting puzzles are not the ones involving "simple" sensations, like thirst hunger, cold, pain, and so on, but rather higher-level mental phenomena, like emotions, judgment, and reasoning. Yet, I think the difference is one of degree of complexity, and basically both types of mental states are part of a general homoeostatic system. Psychologically, the basic phenomenon to consider is a relief and reward seeking circuit whose ultimate role is to keep a certain balance of the organism. Neurologically, this homoeostasis is present at different levels: morpho-functional and biochemical. Azmitia (1999, 2007), for instance, proposes serotonin production and regulation as a basis for the homoeostasis of the nervous system.[2] Serotonin is a powerful chemical to be found both in the brain and in peripheral tissues, acting as neurotransmitter and having a proven role in mental illness, like depression and schizophrenia. It also regulates, among many other processes, sexual behavior and gastrointestinal processes. Most of the quantity of serotonin in the human body, about 95 percent, is present in the guts, but its imbalance in the brain constitutes the biochemical basis of several complex mental phenomena. The way a neurotransmitter like serotonin contributes to constellations of conscious mental states and to complex behavior does not warrant the brain-exclusiveness apparent in the above quotes. Consider the way serotonin is involved in and links somatic with psychiatric illnesses:

> Serotonin has been implicated as an important modulator of cardiovascular and gastrointestinal activity. Although peripheral mechanisms can be expected to predominate, these processes may also partly depend on central serotonin availability. It is thus not surprising that tryptophan has been suggested to link somatic and psychiatric illnesses (Russo et al., 2003). The fact that most serotonin is synthesized and utilized peripherally supports such a notion. (Feenstra and van der Plasse 2010: 253)

More generally, we cannot separate, without loss of explanatory adequacy, hormonal, peripheral nervous and central nervous aspects when it comes to many complex mental phenomena. Consider two examples: aggression and anxiety. Arguably, these phenomena are

---

above is compatible with such a case. I am not saying that a positive blood test is necessary for the judge to exculpate him, but that it would be sufficient.

[2] See also Damasio 2003 and Garcia-Segura 2009.

"higher level" than my example of thirst, and one can think of various ways in which they are relevant to ethical issues. Yet, all these phenomena are, or can easily be understood as, constitutively involving a strong peripheral component.

Aggression. The mental states that ultimately cause aggressive behavior are underlain not only by CNS mechanisms but also by PNS processes, especially those of the Autonomic Nervous System (which plays the central role in "fight-or-flight" responses). Haller et al. emphasize these peripheral aspects:

> Behaviour, including aggressive behaviour, is energy dependent, and therefore requires the rapid mobilisation of energy stores. The peripheral catecholamines [*e.g., hormones like dopamine and adrenalin, N.A.*] play an important role in ensuring the energetic backgrounds of behaviour.... Metabolic preparation for fights has been shown in rodents and this may be under the control of peripheral catecholamines. (1997: 86)

> Noradrenergic activation related to social challenge affects aggression on three different levels, the hormonal level, the sympathetic autonomous nervous system, and the CNS, in different, but functionally synergistic ways. (1997: 92)

Is it especially useful, either from a philosophical or from a neuroscientific point of view, to try to separate the CNS components in these processes and to try to argue that it is only the brain which is the seat of conscious states that cause aggressive behavior? I don't see much sense in such an endeavor. It appears rather that the conscious states are worth being taken as embodied both in the brain and the autonomous PNS, as well as at the hormonal level. Anger, fear, subjective perception of a threat should rather be considered as partly embodied in such peripheral processes, or the constant interaction among hormonal, PNS and CNS events. Finally, when it comes to ethical issues, for instance, pharmacological control of aggressive behavior, intervention at the hormonal, PNS, and CNS levels should be considered equally relevant.

Anxiety and psychosurgery. The term "psychosurgery" refers to surgical intervention on a subject with the goal of treating some mental disorder. Although popular among professionals between the 1930s and 1950s, it rapidly fell into disrepute, mainly because new drugs were discovered and developed, which were more efficacious than surgery, and, more importantly, because of disturbing ethical implications of such procedures, as perceived by both professionals and the public. Lobotomy, a procedure by which all connections of the prefrontal cortex with the rest of the brain are destroyed, used to be, for a long time, the typical image of psycho-surgery in popular culture. Lobotomy was considered a "therapy" for extreme cases of psychopathy, by rendering the subjects "easier to handle." Many lobotomized subjects become permanently inca-pacitated and lose most of their mental lives; they become demented and docile.

Although very controversial, some forms of psychosurgery have known a recent revival. Surgical intervention on the brain is nowa-days always done at the level of the limbic system (the one respon-sible for the regulation of emotions), as a treatment of extreme forms of disorders like depression, which endanger the subject's life or involves a high risk of self-injury by the subject.

However, not all psychosurgery is done at the level of the CNS. Endoscopic sympathetic blocking (ESB), or *sympathectomy*, is a surgical procedure done at the level of the sympathetic division autonomic nervous system, by which the main sympathetic nerve trunk that connects the CNS to the periphery is either sectioned or blocked by the application of a clamp. It is not a surgery of the brain, but of the PNS. Recently, it has been used in the treatment of anxiety disorders and that of some symptoms of schizophrenia (Telaranta 2003). As anxiety disorder involves abnormal emotional regulation, it is no wonder the autonomic PNS, as well as the endo-crine system which produces and circulates hormones, are as rele-vant as the brain when it comes to treatment options and the connected potential ethical implications. Of course, one can always insist, saying: "ultimately, it is the brain we want to intervene upon, albeit indirectly, by disturbing the functioning of the PNS and the endocrine system." I think this reaction is likely to come from those philosophers who usually take the question of where exactly experience is located too seriously and also think that it must be in a well-circumscribed place in the brain. However, it is, from an empirical point of view, not so important to settle such a metaphysical question, much less so to somehow assume, a priori, that experiences have to have a definite "place in the brain." To take our example of anxiety disorder, it involves pathological levels of some emotions, like fear and worry. But it also involves somatic symptoms, like sweating, heart racing, blushing, shortness of breath, stomach ache, trembling, and others, which are manifesta-tions of the autonomic PNS and the endocrine system. Now, you could consider these manifestations, which also have a sensory component, as merely causes of the phenomenal qualities associated to these emotional states, but you could equally consider them as constitutive components of those states.[3]

In any case, in what follows I will try to offer a fresh look at some ethical issues where I think that some novel points can be made based on taking the PNS as seriously as the brain is usually taken. I will consider two issues, each discussed in a separate section: the morally right time to abort a fetus and the issue of whether it is permissible or even obligatory to satisfy the request by Body Integrity Identity Disorder patients to have one of their limbs amputated.

I. Abortion: Thick Potentiality

The literature on the ethical problems related to abortion is quantitatively considerable and wide-ranging in terms of the disciplines involved. It is a topic that could hardly be addressed with any seriousness if one decides to limit argumentation to purely conceptual, a priori, "armchair reasoning." The issue is further complicated by the political factor. Even if the issue of the moral permissibility or otherwise of abortion, at some stage or other of gestation, were tractable by armchair reflection alone, there would still be further disagreement about whether the concepts and analyses proposed are politically colored and motivated. There is likely no solution to this problem that is to satisfy all the relevant constraints: a priori

---

[3] Similar considerations would apply to other ethically relevant cases, for instance, the issue of whether chemical castration of recidivist paraphiliac sexual offenders is ethically acceptable. Chemical castration consist of reducing the level of circulating, free testosterone, the main male androgenic hormone, to virtually zero in the subject, thus killing off the sexual drive, the occurrence of sexual fantasizing, as well as the capacity to engage in sexual intercourse in males. Typically, one of the arguments against the ethicalness of chemical castration is that it affects the very core of personhood, part of which is sexual drive and sexual fantasizing, by indirectly acting on the CNS (Stinneford 2005). But, I think, an equally good argument could be that it interferes with basic homeostatic processes of the organism, regulated by the autonomic PNS and the endocrine system. Maybe the public tends to agree with chemical castration of sexual offenders, especially of pedophiles, not only because of the terrible acts they have committed but also because there is a hidden prejudice that the "real or genuine person" of such offenders is a mind that has been captured by hormones, and that there is nothing wrong in "killing off these hormones and liberate the person from their vicious influence." This is only a guess; it would be interesting to investigate these attitudes toward chemical castration empirically. I say it is a prejudice because part of what it means to be a mentally healthy and well adapted individual involves a huge influence of the hormonal component, not only testosterone, but all other hormones, and, as a matter of fact, sexual offenders *do not* have abnormally high levels of free testosterone (Rösler and Witztum 2000).

acceptability, empirical adequacy, and political neutrality. Nevertheless, some progress can be made at least on the first two aspects.

The nervous system is most relevant to the issue in certain arguments and less so in others. This is why I will not discuss, for example, the arguments for the view that even if the fetus is a person, women's choice of aborting it is morally permissible.[4] The reason is that it looks plausible that if facts about the nervous system of the fetus are relevant, then they are most relevant when one accepts the premise that if a fetus is a person, then it is prima facie not always morally permissible to destroy it, because then the main question is what makes a fetus of a certain age a person. And here most philosophers and scientist would agree that what we are searching for is empirical information about the nervous system. However, conceptual analysis must also be employed when it comes to the notion of a person.

Some philosophers are tempted to start with a discussion of metaphysical views about what a person is and then, after choosing the best metaphysics, apply the result to the moral and legal domains of rights of persons.[5] However, others are skeptical about whether metaphysics has such a primordial conceptual role, and consider that ethics is largely independent of the underlying metaphysics of persons.[6]

Yet, a third view that one can take is that some ethical intuitions about the notion of a person must come first, from which the rudiments of the most plausible metaphysics can be extracted, after which further elaboration of the metaphysics, together with empirical data, will determine the ultimate ethical view about the particular issue, namely the morality of abortion. This is the strategy I will adopt in what follows.

Let us start with the question of what is it about a healthy adult human, anyone we come across on the street, in a restaurant, and so on, that makes us think that it would be wrong to kill her because of a right to life that that human possesses. It looks like, from the point of view of the basis of a right to life, the person typically has (and definitely has the capacity of forming) desires, plans for the immediate or more distant future, is aware of herself, of the world, and of her interactions with the world. In other words, the person is

[4] The classic article where this argument is discussed is in Judith Jarvis Thomson (1971). See also Frances Kamm (1992), for further discussion.

[5] For instance, Parfit 1986.

[6] For instance, Conee 1999.

someone who has a concept of self as a continuant entity, with past experiences and potential future, and views herself as distinct from anyone else, with particular plans and desires. Call this complex of mental properties "self-consciousness." Indeed, Michael Tooley (1972, 1984) proposed such a notion of a person as the only notion that could serve as ground for the right not to have one's life terminated without one's consent. Peter Singer (1993) is also happy to adopt this notion as relevant for the issue of abortion, and, like Tooley, is ready to go where the argument appears to lead, namely, that infanticide (i.e., killing a newborn) is morally acceptable, if it is done before a certain age at which the baby acquires the properties to qualify as a person in the above sense (according to the empirical data they rely on, before one month since birth). It would be an ad hominem to say that Tooley and Singer are politically motivated in coming up with a concept of a person that would morally justify abortion at any prenatal stage and are ready to bite the bullet and accept that it is not intrinsically morally wrong to kill a baby if it is young enough. Yet, both of them explicitly assert that their goal is to justify the "liberal position" on abortion (or rather to offer a *coherent* liberal position), so they would not take the claim that their concepts are politically motivated as an accusation.

When it comes to the idea that it is not intrinsically morally wrong to kill an infant, if, for example, her parents decide so, my guess is that not many people except Tooley and Singer would be undisturbed, to say the least. Singer, for instance, is aware that most people find his conclusion appalling, but he insists that people's view must be challenged. In his tackling these intuitions on the part of most people, he puts on paper some truly fallacious pieces of reasoning. One such piece is that our intuition in this case comes from the Christian tradition, so it is presumably not pre-theoretical or pure in some sense. But why should it depend on what its origins are whether the intuition qualifies to be taken seriously and used in our moral reasoning or not? Then he argues that Ancient cultures, including the highly developed Greek and Roman civilizations, practiced infanticide as a means for population control and eugenics, and that someone like Plato, Aristotle, or Seneca certainly were not less morally evolved than we are today. Here is a quote from Singer ([1993] 2011: 173):

> We might think that we are just more 'civilised' than these 'primitive' peoples. But it is not easy to feel confident that we are more civilised than the best Greek and Roman moralists. It was not just the Spartans who exposed their infants on hillsides: both Plato and Aristotle

recommended the killing of deformed infants. Romans like Seneca, whose compassionate moral sense strikes the modern reader (or me, anyway) as superior to that of the early and mediaeval Christian writers, also thought infanticide the natural and humane solution to the problem posed by sick and deformed babies. The change in Western attitudes to infanticide since Roman times is, like the doctrine of the sanctity of human life of which it is a part, a product of Christianity. Perhaps it is now possible to think about these issues without assuming the Christian moral framework that has, for so long, prevented any fundamental reassessment.

Well, I don't know whether Singer would also accept Aristotle's explicitly derogatory view of women (and Plato's to a lesser extent), or Plato's ideas to the effect that uneducated people should not have any say in politics, and other such views, just because they had "such a compassionate moral sense." In any case, unless his "liberalism" allows him to accept these, Singer will have to bite many other bullets, in order to end up with a coherent view.[7]

Be that as it may, I still think that the above notion of a person is the relevant one when it comes to trying to answer the question of what makes a *healthy adult human* qualify as a person in a way that confers the right not to be killed without consent. Where I differ from Tooley and Singer is that I don't think that it really follows that infants and, as I will argue, fetuses after a certain age are morally acceptable to be killed, everything else being equal. The argument for this that I will employ is a so-called "potentiality argument." Now, potentiality arguments have forcefully been tackled by philosophers interested in defending the liberal position about abortion, and I think that the intuitions behind the criticism of the potentiality arguments are very powerful. However, the potentiality argument I want to put forward is very different from what has been proposed so far. The old potentiality argument goes something like the following:

(1) Given the biological laws of nature, the zygote/embryo/fetus would develop (has the potential to develop) into a full-fledged person, with experiences, self-consciousness and plans for the future.

(2) The potentiality of an entity to become a person raises the moral status of that entity to that of a person.

(3) Hence, the zygote/embryo/fetus has the moral status of a person.

---

[7]My guess is that most of the liberals about abortion would definitely find the moral acceptability of killing newborn infants appalling. I base my judgment on my own case, as well as that of most of my friends, who happen to be liberal about abortion.

(4) It is morally wrong to destroy an entity with the moral status of a person.

(5) Hence, it is morally wrong to destroy the zygote/embryo/fetus.

The argument has been the target of criticism and even mockery because most people have the intuition that, for instance, the zygote and the embryo do not have any moral status, yet if premise 2 in the argument is right, then we should think that they do have the moral status of a person due to their potentiality in developing into a person. Here are a couple of quotes that point out, correctly in my opinion, that mere potentiality, or what I will call "thin potentiality," should not be taken as conferring moral properties on the entity who possesses this potentiality. One is from Gazzaniga (2006: 143):

> The potentiality argument is similar, in that it views having the potential to develop into a human being as conferring equal status to that of a human being. I have made the point elsewhere (Gazzaniga 2005) that this is akin to saying that a Home Depot do-it-yourself store is the same as 100 houses because it holds that potential. The main problem, and one that neuroscience cannot ignore, is that this belief makes no sense. How can a biological entity that has no nervous system be a moral agent?

The other is from Tooley (1972: 60–61), where he considers an imaginary case of a kitten potentially becoming a person:

> My argument against the potentiality principle can now be stated. Suppose at some future time a chemical were to be discovered which when injected into the brain of a kitten would cause the kitten to develop into a cat possessing a brain of the sort possessed by humans, and consequently into a cat having all the psychological capabilities characteristic of adult humans. Such cats would be able to think, to use language, and so on. Now it would surely be morally indefensible in such a situation to ascribe a serious right to life to members of the species *Homo sapiens* without also ascribing it to cats that have undergone such a process of development: there would be no morally significant differences....
>
> Secondly, it would not be seriously wrong to refrain from injecting a newborn kitten with the special chemical, and to kill it instead....
>
> Thirdly, in view of the symmetry principle, if it is not seriously wrong to refrain from initiating such a causal process, neither is it seriously wrong to interfere with such a process....
>
> But if it is not seriously wrong to destroy an injected kitten which will naturally develop the properties that bestow a right to life, neither can it be seriously wrong to destroy a member of *Homo sapiens* which lacks such properties, but will naturally come to have them. The potentialities are the same in both cases.

What these authors are right about is that mere potentiality cannot intuitively constitute the ground for moral status. Let me introduce my notion of *thin potentiality*, and then the notion of *thick potentiality*.

Thin potentiality:
For some property F and time t, x has *thin potential* at t to become an F iff (i) at t, x is not F, and (ii) there is a causal process C, such that if C is in place at t, then at some later time t^*, x is F.

Gazzaniga's house-building process and the materials in the home depot qualify as the causal process C and the individual x, respectively, in our definition, so that x being F signifies the materials being put together as houses. Mutatis mutandis for Tooley's kitten. The counterintuitiveness of this notion of potentiality as used in the argument against abortion resides in that condition (ii) is so permissive as to always make it the case that even though condition (i) holds, that is, x is not F, the entity under scrutiny, x, would qualify as similar enough in some important way to an F. For instance, an extrinsic, artificial causal process, like injecting Tooley's chemical into a kitten, qualifies as a referent for C. Also, even if the causal process is intrinsic to x and natural, it may involve some changes to x that would be equivalent to x ceasing to be the kind that it was at the time the causal process started. I take the developmental causal process from fertilized egg to fetal organism, for example, in humans and other vertebrates, as one that brings about the egg going out of existence, since an egg is not an organism.

Let me now introduce another notion, that of thick potentiality.

Thick potentiality:
For some property F and time t, x has *thick potential* at t to become an F iff (i) at t, x is G and not F, (ii) there is a causal process C, such that if C is in place at t, then at some later time t^*, x is F, and (iii) F is a degree of G.

Putting aside Tooley's kitten for now, if we consider again Gazzaniga's case with the home depot, it is apparent that the property of being a house is not a degree of any property that the house-components sitting in the depot possess, either individually or collectively. Maybe in the case of being a house it is anyway hard to think of a property that would be a lesser degree of it, but other examples abound. Consider the property of an apple or of certain kinds of cured cheese of *being ripe*. Suppose it takes a month for an apple, or three months for a blue cheese, to ripen. If in the middle of these periods we ask whether the apple, or the cheese, is ripe the answer is no, but they are in a state of ripening, which means that if the causal process that is active at that time continues, their becoming ripe is a matter of the same kinds of properties that they possess becoming more intense on some scale of intensity. For example, the Gorgonzola cheese might not be ripe yet after a couple of weeks of curing, but the properties that make it count as ripe at three months of curing are already present to a lesser extent in it at two weeks: firmness, pungency, blueness, fattiness. The piece of curing organic matter is not yet a piece of Gorgonzola, yet attaining its "gorgonzo-lahood" is matter of that piece's properties increasing in intensity.

My claims will be that (a) newborn babies, as well as fetuses after a certain age, do have a thick potential to become persons, that is, self-conscious beings, and that (b) thick potentiality is sufficient for the right to life. A corollary of (a) will be that fetuses before the relevant age, and a fortiori zygotes and embryos, do not have a thick potentiality to become human. At the end of the section, after I also present empirical evidence for my preferred cut-off time in fetal development that separates right and wrong when it comes to destroying the fetus, as well as for my conceptual claims when they are relevant, I will also offer a reply to Tooley's case with the kitten. As we shall see, the PNS will be relevant when it comes to the empirical question about the cut-off time.

First, let me offer a culinary analogy that will help establish claim (b). Here is a typical muffin recipe that you can easily find on the internet:

Ingredients:
1 medium egg, beaten
2 cups of flour
3/4 cup of milk
1/2 cup of sugar
1/2 cup of oil
3 teaspoons of baking powder
1/2 teaspoon of almond extract
1/4 teaspoon of cinnamon
1/4 teaspoon of nutmeg
1/8 teaspoon of salt

Instructions:
   Mix together the egg, milk, oil, and almond extract. In another bowl, mix together the flour, sugar, baking powder, nutmeg, cinnamon, and salt. Mix the two mixtures. Bake at 390°F for about 15 minutes.

Suppose that you want to surprise your partner, who is on the way home, by making muffins. You prepare all the ingredients on a table and you are ready to start the process as described in the instructions above. You are lucky, you say to yourself, because you have exactly the quantities of ingredients that you need in order to have the muffins ready by the time she/he arrives. Your small child is playing around in the kitchen and manages to pour the contents of your bag of flour into the sink, thus preventing you from making the muffins. Did your child manage to destroy the muffins? Although the flour is essential to the recipe (no flower, no muffin), I don't think we would normally and literally say that the muffins got destroyed. Now consider the following cases:

A. Your child pours the milk
B. You manage to make the mix of egg, milk, oil and almond extract, but your child throws it in the garbage.
C. You manage to pour the final mixture into small muffin cups in a baking tray and then leave the tray in the preheated oven, but after a couple of minutes of baking, your child takes the tray from the oven and throws it out of the window.

In the first two cases we would not normally and literally say that your child managed to destroy *the muffins*; the first case is analogous to that of pouring the flour into the sink, whereas in the second case we would merely say that your child managed to destroy the mix. However, once the mix is in the process of baking in the hot oven, in muffin cups arranged on a baking tray, it is plausible to literally say that your child has destroyed your muffins, even though, strictly speaking, it is not yet a something that you would eat *and claim to have eaten a muffin*. The point is even better supported if we return to our Gorgonzola cheese. Even though if you eat the piece of cheese after two weeks of curing, you wouldn't, strictly speaking, say that you have eaten Gorgonzola, yet, if someone were to dump it, you would say that that person destroyed your Gorgonzola. The relation between the half-baked muffin mix and the muffin, as well as the relation between the half-cured Gorgonzola mass and the piece of ripe Gorgonzola is one of thick potentiality. At the same time, neither destroying the milk as such, nor destroying the apple seed as such count as destroying some cheese or an apple, respectively, because the properties these have are not plausibly degrees of *gorgonzolahood* and *applehood*, respectively.

What characterizes the relation of thick potentiality is our willingness to assert that losing the developing relatum is tantamount to having lost the relatum that would have developed from the former, and what grounds this assertion is that the properties in virtue of which the potential relatum counts as developed are higher degrees of the properties that the actual relatum already possesses. A good heuristics to test our intuition about whether x being G is related by thick potentiality to x being F is to ask whether it is the mere continuation of the same processes that make x being G that would make x being F later. The relation is that of thick potentiality iff the answer to this question is positive. Informally, the question is: for some x that is G, does adding the same kind of stuff (increasing the magnitude of G) to x make it F?

For example, the process of making Gorgonzola starts with some bacteria being added to some quantity of whole cow's milk. Does adding more of the same stuff—that is, continuing to add bacteria to the milk—make it Gorgonzola after a while? The answer is no; merely adding more bacteria would actually spoil the milk. The second stage is that of fermentation, after the right quantity of bacteria has been added. Does adding more of the same stuff—that is, continuing the fermentation process—make it Gorgonzola after a while? Not yet. There is a stage of removing whey via the process of curdling. More fermentation without curdling does not result in anything like a cheese whatsoever. The only stage at which we have thick potentiality is after the whey has been removed and now the curd starts the process of aging. At this point the answer to our question is yes: the curd becoming Gorgonzola is a matter of the curd aging for long enough; it is a *degree* of aging.

Based on the above analogies we can say that, when it comes to destroying some G that has the thick potential to become an F, it is intuitively justified to think of the destruction of the G as if it were the destruction of an F, even though G is distinct from F. So if it is morally wrong to destroy an F, then this moral wrongness will be transferred to the destruction of the G. This means that for whichever entity during the post-conception development has a thick potential to become a person in Tooley and Singer's sense, that is, a self-conscious being, it is morally wrong to destroy that entity.

As it happens, I think that both newborn babies and fetuses at a certain age have properties that make them possess the thick potential to become persons, so it is morally wrong to kill those fetuses and babies. This is my claim (a), which I would like to argue for in what follows.

As we agreed before, the complex of mental properties that make someone a person is self-consciousness. The mental properties that enter this complex are states, capacities, and dispositions (e.g., the state of being concerned about one's own future, as well as the capacity and the disposition to become so concerned). Nowadays, most of us are implicitly or explicitly naturalists, so we believe that the instantiation of the mental properties that enter the complex of self-consciousness is entirely and exclusively dependent on some facts about the nervous system. Indeed, we can be more precise and assert, based on empirical evidence, that most probably self-consciousness, because it is a relatively late phenomenon in child development, is connected to the development of higher areas of processing in the neocortex and/or thalamus. To give one example, self-reflection, that is the psychological activity of thinking about oneself, which undoubtedly we would include under our general category of self-consciousness, and hence personhood, is likely to be ultimately essentially realized in the medial prefrontal and posterior cingulate cortex; both lesion studies (Damasio et al. 1990) and fMRI imaging (Johnson et al. 2002) point in this direction.

Now, it looks likes self-reflection and all other components of what we consider relevant to self-consciousness, and therefore to personhood, once we focus on the neural basis of these, are simply higher degrees of simpler or more primitive and evolutionarily older such nervous system structures and functions. Self-consciousness is, from a naturalistic point of view (in this case neurobiological), not more than a degree of sophistication of neural processes. The emergence of self-conscious states is not a drastic, extravagant, earth-shaking phenomenon.

Not everyone is, of course, a naturalist; someone could, maybe even coherently, believe that something like the truly autonomous immaterial soul emerges when the brain contains the structural-functional grounds for self-consciousness. However, such a view, besides being quite unbelievable a priori, is hard to ever be justified by empirical data. Furthermore, virtually everyone with a minimal willingness to avoid dogma and prejudice in the abortion debate would be reluctant to base their views on such extravagant metaphysics or anything similar, like some religious doctrine or other.

So what could be the cutoff point in the development of a fetus after which it counts as having the thick potential for personhood? The most general mental property that we usually take as morally relevant is *sentience*. Although it does not appear as right to say that self-consciousness is a higher degree of sentience per se, it is not far-fetched to think of the phenomenal and the functional properties

associated with self-consciousness as a higher degree of the phenomenal and functional properties associated with experiencing the
outer environment. If it turns out that fetuses of a certain age do
possess some degree of sentience, then thereby they possess the
rudiments of personhood, hence they have the thick potential to
become persons, hence they have moral status of a person, even
though they are not yet full-fledged persons. There are many empirical studies that indicate that newborn infants, as well as full-term
fetuses, that is, fetuses who are developed enough for life outside the
womb (roughly after 37 weeks from conception), do possess sentience in the form of sensorimotor capacities (e.g., capacity to feel
pain, to hear, to smell, etc.), as well as the relevant behavioral dispositions. Furthermore, even some higher cognitive capacities are present in the fetus and the newborn infant, like memory. Newborn
babies also develop, within days, the capacity to discriminate
between fragments of speech from different linguistic families and
prefer to listen to their own native language, thus showing a very
early linguistic capacity.[8]

The main question now is: What is the earliest time in the development of a fetus at which it possesses at least one of the mental
properties that would make it possess a thick potential to become a
person? This question has not been definitively answered, as neuroscientists tend to disagree about which aspect of the development of
the nervous system is relevant to consider. There are several authors
who opt for midgestation (20 weeks) as the relevant point when sentience starts, and their argument is that at that point there is EEG
and fMRI evidence that cortical or cortico-thalamic connections
become active. Here are a couple of quotes relevant to this point and
to what I am going to say about fetal sentience in reaction to this
thalamo-cortico-centrism:

> When the fetal human might begin to experience discomfort and pain,
> to know hurt, is a question whose answer is tied to our understanding
> of adult pain. The answer would seem to turn on whether there can be
> anything like the affective dimension of pain ('it hurts') without corti-
> cal participation. Ralston (1984) has reviewed what is known about the
> pathways linking peripheral pain receptors with the central nervous
> system. He finds evidence (in monkeys and other species) that
> somatosensory neurons of the neocortex respond to noxious stimuli

[8]For a summary of all these findings and the relevant bibliography, the reader is
encouraged to consult Lagercrantz and Changeux (2009).

and he concludes that "it does not appear necessary to postulate a sub-cortical mechanism for appreciation of pain" (p. 189). *For Ralston, 'it hurts' is a neocortical state*, if his assessment of the scientific findings is correct, the fetal human cannot experience hurt before the thalamo-cortical connection is made (at mid-gestation), since the noxious stim-ulus pathways pass through the thalamus." (Flower 1985: 247) (emphasis added)

The next quote is more recent and is from a paper synthesizing the results on fetal pain research:

> Pain perception requires conscious recognition or awareness of a nox-ious stimulus. Neither withdrawal reflexes nor hormonal stress responses to invasive procedures prove the existence of fetal pain, *because they can be elicited by nonpainful stimuli and occur without conscious cortical processing*. Fetal awareness of noxious stimuli requires functional thalamocortical connections. Thalamocortical fibers begin appearing between 23 to 30 weeks' gestational age, while electroencephalography suggests the capacity for functional pain per-ception in preterm neonates probably does not exist before 29 or 30 weeks. (Lee et al. 2005: 947) (emphasis added)

What I find interesting is that in both quotes the argument against situating pain states before midgestation is simply the assumption that it must be a cortical or cortico-thalamic state, but there is no further argument as about why it is only the cortex that can be the basis of pain. In the first quote we come across the idea that we need to ensure that the "affective dimension of pain" is present in a fetus in order to be sure that pain is present in it, and that this affective dimension requires cortical activity. But what is the evidence that it requires cortical activity? Well, the evidence is always partly behav-ioral, when the subject of pain can report her discomfort. The fact that a fetus *cannot report* does not normally mean that we should exclude that it is ever in the sensory state of pain. But I find espe-cially prejudiced and fallacious the next argument, part of which appears as the emphasized fragment in the second quote. It says that behavioral and hormonal response to noxious stimulation does not count as evidence of pain because such responses can be elicited by other types of stimuli and can occur without "conscious cortical processing." A first point to be made is that, by analogy, my taking a painkiller is not evidence of my having a headache, because this type of behavior could be elicited while I am sleeping or under the influence of hallucinogenic drugs.

However, more importantly, in considering these pieces of reasoning as a form of bias favoring the cortex, I am not merely putting
forward another, anti-cortical bias. In a recent paper, Bjorn Merker
(2007) offers plenty of empirical evidence to challenge this cortico-
centrism. One of the most powerful pieces of evidence presented by
Merker is that of decorticated newborn humans who can't even be
judged as defective from a sensorimotor perspective in the first year
of their lives. After this first year they miss several developmental
landmarks and become severely disabled. However, with proper
treatment and care:

> These children are not only awake and often alert, but show respon-
> siveness to their surroundings in the form of emotional or orienting
> reactions to environmental events, most readily to sounds, but also to
> salient visual stimuli (optic nerve status varies widely in hydranen-
> cephaly, discussed further on). They express pleasure by smiling and
> laughter, and aversion by "fussing," arching of the back and crying (in
> many gradations), their faces being animated by these emotional states.
> A familiar adult can employ this responsiveness to build up play
> sequences predictably progressing from smiling, through giggling, to
> laughter and great excitement on the part of the child. The children
> respond differentially to the voice and initiatives of familiars, and show
> preferences for certain situations and stimuli over others, such as a
> specific familiar toy, tune, or video program, and apparently can even
> come to expect their regular presence in the course of recurrent daily
> routines. (Merker 2007: 79)

Similar observations have been made in decorticated rats, who
appear to behave similarly to rats with intact cortex, and can cope
with the learning tasks that normal rats can complete, as well as in
decorticated cats, who are capable of purposefully moving around
and of solving visual discrimination tasks (Merker 2007: 74). These
empirical data also constitute a simple and effective answer to Singer's overconfidence that, for instance, in cases of brainstem activity
without the cortex there is no morally relevant mental activity:

> [I]t is not ethically relevant that there is still some hormonal brain
> function, for hormonal brain function without consciousness cannot
> benefit the patient. Nor can brain-stem function alone benefit the
> patient, in the absence of a cortex. (Singer 2006: 192)

As Merker points it out, the brainstem:

> maintains special connective relations with cortical territories impli-
> cated in attentional and conscious functions, but is not rendered non-
> functional in the absence of cortical input. This helps explain the

purposive, goal-directed behavior exhibited by mammals after experimental decortication, as well as the evidence that children born without a cortex are conscious. (2007: 63)

Consequently, we should not have any qualms about challenging the corticocentrist prejudice and being open to the hypothesis that sentience appears prior to cortical integration. Is it possible to establish this point or period during development? I think we can ask a question of what I would like to call "neurohermeneutics," that is, the interpretive activity having as its subject the meaning or teleology behind neural processes.[9] The simplest forms of conscious, phenomenal states are sensory states, like having a brief feeling of pain or of being touched. The question is, therefore: What does it mean in terms of processes of the nervous system to sense as such? Or: What is the meaning or teleology behind the nervous system being in a state or process of sensing? Given the actual structure of the nervous system of humans and most other vertebrates, the answer will essentially involve the PNS. Structurally, to sense anything presupposes a transmission of electrical impulse from some bodily or external medium to the CNS, and that is always done via the PNS. The first such electrical impulse transmission, therefore, will be possible after the PNS or its rudiments are in place. After this occurs, we can say that the occurrence of more complex sensing, perception, and self-consciousness are a matter of "more of the same stuff going on," that is, phenomena that would connect the first electrical impulse to personhood in terms of thick potentiality. The nervous system of the fetus develops following certain stages: stem cell multiplication, formation of neurons (*neurulation*), neurons self-organizing and occupying their positions in the future brain, axonal growth from the brain towards the peripheral sites (i.e., growth of the PNS), end of axonal growth by the nerves reaching their target organs (e.g., skin, internal organs, other receptors), synaptic development, and finally, further structural development and diversification, for instance, by programmed cell death and generation of new fibers and synapses (Rees and Walker 2001). The structurally relevant stage for our question is when axon growth makes the CNS connect to the external and internal environment via the PNS fibers reaching their targets. If there is electrical activity in the

[9] I am aware that the term "neurohermeneutics" already exists and is used by various people with various meanings, though not much in print. My choice of the term here is based on the meanings of its constituent terms, "hermeneutics" (interpretation) and "neuro-" (related to the nervous system), and is nontechnical.

brain before this moment, that activity is not relevant, because it is, given our neurohermeneutics, not an instance of sensing. Consequently, the birth of consciousness and, hence, the birth of persons in the case of humans, whose early sensing has the thick potential for self-consciousness, is the moment when the first *PNS-mediated signal* reaches the brain. As a matter of fact, I do not know of any study that specifically set this question as a research goal, but in any case such electrical activity occurs well before midgestation. Developmental neurologists using ultrasound established that the first signs of fluent, organized, and recurring motor activity of the human fetus (so-called general movements) occur during week 8 post-conception; the fetus generates spontaneous movements of the extremities and exhibits other behavioral patterns, like startles, hiccups, and yawning (Dalton and Bergenn 2007: 61). At 7.5 weeks, the fetus exhibits whole-body movements away from a stimulus, as observed on a sonogram. Furthermore, at approximately 8 weeks the perioral region (the region around the mouth) responds to tactile stimulation, and by week 14 most of the body is sensitive to touch (Miller et al. 2005: 8).

To summarize the ideas I have argued for, we can say that the time t after which it is morally wrong to kill a fetus is the time at which its nervous system exhibits for the first time a state with thick potential for self-consciousness, that is, a state S such that self-consciousness is, neurologically speaking, a higher degree of S. This state is the first instance of sensing, evidence of which is coherent, organized motor response to stimulation. My argument is not supposed to be taken as saying anything about legal issues about regulating abortion. These issues are more complex than the problem of when the unborn acquires certain properties that make it have a relation of thick potentiality to become a person. During the entire discussion I have presented, the reader is asked to keep in my mind that there is a ceteris paribus caveat, so that my neuroscience based conclusion is merely: *everything else being equal*, it is wrong to destroy the fetus after 8 weeks post-conception. Of course, in reality not everything is equal and it is not only the fetus's nervous development that exhausts the set of factors relevant to the issue of abortion, but also, for example, the weighing of the interests of the fetus and the mother in each specific case. What my argument was rather directed at is the Tooley-Singer type of approach, according to which the liberal view of abortion is incoherent unless it allows infanticide. The liberal view is perfectly compatible with the existence of a cutoff point in time of fetal development before which abortion is morally permissible and after which it is impermissible (ceteris paribus).

Let me end with a rebuttal of Tooley's case with the kitten. Tooley imagines a chemical that could make a kitten develop a human brain and consciousness. So if the kitten is injected with the chemical, it will acquire the potentiality for self-consciousness. Yet, Tooley claims, it is not morally wrong to refrain from injecting the kitten and killing it instead. So, just like it is morally permitted to kill the kitten before it acquires the potentiality to become human, it is also not morally wrong to kill a fetus or a newborn human *before* it becomes self-conscious.

The problem with Tooley's line of thought, however, is that *after* the kitten is injected, it has the thick potential for becoming a person, so it is wrong to kill it. Before it is injected it does not have the thick potential for personhood, so it is not wrong to kill it (if it is done painlessly). What about the fetus? The same reasoning applies, before the fetus has a sensory state, it does not have the thick potential for becoming a person, hence, it is not wrong to kill it. After the first sensory state occurs, the fetus has the thick potential for personhood, so it is wrong to kill it. The kitten case does not show, given our notion of thick potentiality, that it is not wrong to kill fetuses and newborn babies. On the other hand, as long as there is no such chemical, or as long as the kitten is not injected with such a chemical, it is not morally wrong to kill it, because the kitten lacks the thick potential for becoming a person. It lacks such a potential because, as a matter of biology in the actual world, it is naturally impossible for nonhuman animals to develop personhood. In fact, if such a chemical existed, injecting it into a kitten would be tantamount to creating a new species, or a chimera, which we could call *Felis sapiens*. Contrary to its name, it would not belong to the family of felines. This last point is relevant against an idea that Tooley (and Singer) heavily relies on, namely, that the level of consciousness of a human fetus or newborn is the same as that of a nonhuman animal, hence if the fetus and the newborn have the right to live, the same right should be awarded to nonhuman animals. But if I am right in the above analysis, the temporary similarities regarding mental development between humans and nonhumans are irrelevant to the ethical issue. What is relevant is rather whether an organism has the thick potential to become a person, and nonhuman animals lack this potential at any stage of their development, because it is biologically impossible for them to become persons,[10] whereas in the life of a fetus there is a point at which it acquires this thick potential. It is totally irrelevant that when the fetus acquires thick potential for personhood its consciousness is lower in degree or quality than that of any adult vertebrate. What matters is (a) that, unlike these other vertebrates, the conscious fetus is programmed to develop into a person, and (b) that personhood is a higher degree of sentience.[11]

II. Amputation: Peripheral Precedence

The 2003 documentary, *Whole*, directed by Melody Gilbert, presents cases of people with otherwise healthy limbs who become obsessed with the desire to amputate one or more of these limbs. I am not aware of official statistics about the number of such cases, but some authors assert that there are thousands of such "wannabes," that is, subjects who definitely want their limb amputated (Elliott 2003; Bayne and Levy 2005). If the extent of this anomaly is indeed this large, then the question of whether it is ethical for surgeons to respond positively or negatively to amputation requests by these subjects is not merely a question of philosophical scholarly curiosity, but a socially pressing one. However, whereas the desire to have one's limb amputated might have a non-negligible frequency, it is less clear that the psycho-pathological condition for which the ethical question arises in a most subtle way, in the sense of there being intuitions both *pro* and *contra*, namely, Body Integrity Identity Disorder (BIID), is too frequent. Indeed, if one looks at the bibliography on the desire for amputation, one realizes that the articles,

---

[10]There is a body of research on apes and other mammals (dolphins and elephants) that show that these animals do possess some form of self-consciousness (Gallup 1970; Reiss and Marino 2001; Plotnik et al. 2006). If that kind of self-consciousness qualifies for personhood, then these animals will be exceptions to my claim, and they will have the right to live, just like humans.

[11]One could insist at this point that, for all I said, fetuses or infants with brains damaged in such a way that they will not develop self-consciousness are not intrinsically morally wrong to kill. But this does not follow. In fact, when such damage occurs all we can assert is that it is very unlikely that these subjects can develop self-consciousness; we cannot say, unlike in the case of nonhuman animals, that it is *biologically impossible*, given the species we deal with, to develop self-consciousness. We can't know whether in the future new technology and pharmacological development will not be able to rehabilitate such subjects. On the other hand, as I argued above, if such medical development would be able "to make a self-conscious cat," then we would not be dealing with the species *cat* any more, but rather with humans with cat bodies.

both medical and philosophical, on this topic written before 2000 are almost exclusively focused on *apotemnophilia*, the aberrant sexual attraction to amputated bodies, whereas after 2000 most of them deal with BIID.

That the ethical question does arise beyond the usual academic circles is proven by the media attention some such amputations of healthy limbs have received. The case of surgeon Robert Smith, based in Scotland, who had fulfilled two such patients' desire, in 1997 and 1999, was covered in five articles in *The Guardian* during 2000, as well as in other newspapers. The usual reaction to such surgical intervention is negative. The ethical committee of the hospital where Smith worked decided to ban such interventions. Nevertheless, some bioethicists think that a good case can be made when the cause of the desire is BIID rather than other affections that can be involved. For instance, Bayne and Levy (2005) argue that because BIID is not a condition of delusion, like most other possible candidates for the desire, because patients truly feel or experience, that is, at the phenomenal level, that their limb is alien to them, that it is a foreign body attached to the real one, what is relevant when making an ethical choice regarding amputation reduces to the questions of whether the patients are autonomous in their choice and whether they are aware of the possible consequences of such a drastic intervention, that is, whether they are well-informed. Thus, they assert that:

> If the desire for amputation is long-standing, the patient is not psychotic, and he is well aware of the risks and consequences, surgery is ethically permissible because it will prevent many BIID patients from injuring or killing themselves. (Bayne and Levy 2005: 79)

Similarly, other philosophers argue that it is important to recognize and try to imagine what it is like to be a wannabe, and not be influenced by either media sensationalism, by immediate ordinary intuitions, or by prior ethical doctrines, and realize that there is a case to be made for elective surgery (Bridy 2004; Tomasini 2006).

It is important to distinguish, following Bayne and Levy, between cases in which the desire to have one's limb amputated is based on delusional belief and those when this is not the case. In the medical literature several types of causes of the amputation desire have been hypothesized and described, and it looks as though BIID is the only one type of cause that would qualify as justifying the decision to amputate. For instance, in some cases the patient suffers from Body Dismorphic Disorder (BDD), a condition of delusional belief, when the patient develops an obsession that some body part of hers, with a slight defect, is ugly and needs to be removed. As several authors have pointed out (Crerand et al. 2006; Dyl et al. 2006) the condition persists even after cosmetic medical treatment, and sometimes the symptoms exacerbate. In some other cases, the main cause for the amputation desire is apotemnophilia, that is, a paraphilia (aberrant sexual desire), characterized by attraction felt toward people with amputated limbs, as well as fetishism with respect to objects like wheelchairs or crutches. According to psychiatrist Michael First (2004), who coined the name BIID, apotemnophilia and BIID are strongly correlated. Nevertheless, BIID is a different affection, with different psychological features. Whereas apotemnophilia and BDD, when they are exclusively responsible for the amputation desire, are relatively easy to reject as justifying amputation, because they are based on either delusional beliefs (BDD) or sexual aberration (apotemnophilia), BIID has a different status, or at least the few philosophers who have discussed the issue think so. Patients with BIID typically assert that they do not feel their limb as their own, so, the argument goes, since feeling one's body part as one's own or not is a matter of subjective phenomenology, and since one cannot be (completely) wrong about how one feels, the patient's belief that forms the basis of their amputation desire is not delusional. So the amputation desire of BIID patients who do not happen to also suffer from conditions like BDD and apotemnophilia, or some other paraphilia, would prima facie qualify to be seriously considered to be satisfied by surgical intervention.

The argument has as one of its premises that patients do feel that one of their limbs is alien to them. However, this is a contentious claim. As Bayne and Levy themselves remark (2005: 76), it is unlikely that BIID patients' mismatch is between the body schema and the body, but merely between the body *image* and the body (see our chapter 7 for the distinction). Proof for this claim is that BIID patients do not have a peripherally manifested dysfunction; they use their unwanted limb in the normal functional ways. This means that what patients refer to as "feeling one's limb as alien" is not proprioceptive but cognitive. It is rather a way they can't resist *thinking* about their problematic limb.

It could be argued that there are other cases of surgery requests that were initially controversial because they were based on an identity disorder with a strong cognitive component, but nowadays such surgical interventions are accepted. The relevant such case is Gender Identity Disorder (GID) of transgender and transsexual individuals, which can be treated by sex change surgery. Indeed, both some medical doctors and some BIID patients themselves tend to make an analogy between sex change surgery and amputation. Here is a fragment from a letter to *The Guardian*, by surgeon Richard Green, dated February 3, 2000:

> As head of the NHS sex-change programme, the furor of healthy limb amputation seems to me a case of deja-vu (Healthy limbs cut off at patients' request, February 1). In 1966, at the University of California, I studied physicians' attitudes toward sex-change surgery. The majority preferred that desperate patients commit suicide rather than undergo genital surgery. Amputating healthy sexual organs was characterised as surgical mutilation and psychiatric collusion with delusion. Only after years of futile attempts by psychiatrists to make transsexuals accept their birth sex was surgical treatment begun. The rationale for the 1966 programme at the Johns Hopkins Hospital in the US was "if we cannot change the mind to fit the body, then we must change the body to fit the mind." ... Half of the world lives as men and half as women. There is no large population content to be missing a leg. There is as yet no substantial body of psychiatric treatment results from attempts to cure this disorder of body image to match the well-documented futility of curing transsexualism.

Similarly, on the weblog dedicated to BIID, *transabled.org*, authored by subjects suffering from the condition, one finds articles where the argument is that the amputation desire should be approached like the sex change desire in the case of transsexuals. Sex change operations are nowadays accepted as a way to solve the problem of GID, so it is only a matter of time for amputation in cases of BIID to become an acceptable intervention.

However, there is an important difference between the effects of these two types of surgery. Whereas amputation leads to dysfunction, namely, it brings about a motor disability, sex change surgery is considered reconstructive. Indeed, alternative names for this type of operation are "gender *reassignment* surgery," "genital *reconstruction* surgery," "sex *affirmation* surgery," and "sex *realignment* surgery." The typical patient requesting such operation is a male who wants to become female. The patients' desire does not reduce to the idea of having his penis removed and neither does surgery exhaust the entire treatment procedure, but it is accompanied by hormone replacement therapy. In other words, patients do not desire a sexual dysfunction or disability, but a gender reassignment of normal sexual functions. Moreover, both BIID patients themselves, on *transabled.org*, and very recently some core researchers of the phenomenon

(First and Fisher 2012) have argued for the definition of BIID as "the persistent desire to acquire a physical disability." Under this new definition, it is not only the desire for amputation of limbs that is relevant, but various other desires that patients do express, like the desire to become blind, deaf, or paralyzed. For instance, the desire to become blind can hardly be considered analogous to the desire for amputation, if what one takes to explain the latter is some discrepancy between the body map in the brain and the body itself. Indeed, many BIID patients, when they first develop the symptoms, usually in adolescence, start by pretending to be disabled, for instance, by limping or using a wheelchair. The psychological explanation for this urge is a need for more attention and affection.

What can we make of all this? I think it is useful to distinguish two questions. One is whether it is *intrinsically* wrong or not to satisfy a request for amputation or for sectioning some peripheral nerves, or the spinal cord, with the goal of rendering someone paraplegic, blind, or deaf. The other question is whether it is wrong or not *overall* to satisfy such requests. The answer to the second question is more relevant for practical purposes, but answering the first one is a necessary step in order to even get a positive answer to the second off the ground. If it is not intrinsically wrong to satisfy one's desire to be mutilated, then, of course, there might by other reasons not to do it, but, at the same time, extrinsic considerations, those related to various information about the context (e.g., the likely harmful consequences of a positive or negative answer to the request) might sanction such a surgical intervention as desirable.

Bayne and Levy offer several arguments for the permissibility of amputation, but one of them seems to me the most elaborate, namely, the argument from autonomy. They argue that at least in the case of BIID patients, we have agents who are completely aware of the consequences of such an intervention, they are autonomous agents, hence, their view about their own good should be given due respect. Moreover, Bayne and Levy think that in an important sense their limbs are not healthy, so in that sense these patients are not delusional:

> Perhaps BIID involves a similar form of nondelusional somatic alienation. If so, then there might be a very real sense in which the limb in question—or at least, the neuronal representation of it—is not healthy. (2005: 77)

> Are wannabes with BIID delusional? We have already suggested that they are not. Although wannabes seem not to experience parts of their

body as their own, they do not go on to form the corresponding belief that it is alien. The wannabe with BIID clearly recognizes that the leg is hers: she does not identify it as someone else's leg, nor does she attempt to throw it out of bed, in the way that patients with somatoparaphrenia sometimes do. (2005: 81)

There is a problem, however. If BIID includes subjects who want to become blind, then there is little reason to think that their eyes, or the neural representation of them, are not healthy. Furthermore, as Bayne and Levy themselves note (2005: 76, 78), BIID patients seem not to be bothered by wearing prostheses after the surgery. So it is likely that not even the neural representation of the leg, or eyes, and so on can be said to be unhealthy in some way. The real desire seems to be not to get rid of a limb per se, but to acquire some disability. Which disability subjects want to acquire varies from person to person. So I think that ultimately the desire for amputation is neurologically speaking grounded in and sustained by higher-level, cognitive-affective facts, and not by lower-level, somatosensory facts.

I would like to put forward a principle, which I call "peripheral precedence" (PP), based on which we can judge cases like the amputation request. The principle could be formulated as follows:

(PP) Given a request, R, for some medical intervention, I, by a patient, P, in order to satisfy a perceived rational need, N, of P's, such that if R were satisfied, some otherwise healthy part, S, of P's nervous system would, as a result of I, be completely destroyed or completely lose its function, satisfying R is morally permissible only if (a) I is the only type of intervention that is likely to satisfy N, and (b) the neural basis of N is at the same level or more peripheral than S, relative to the highest processing areas of P's nervous system, above a certain threshold for S to count as fulfilling a non-negligible function for P's organism.

The principle, of course, is to be understood as applicable to the actual world, given what we know about and the way we think about the nervous systems of actual humans. Crucial here is the empirically supported assumption that by "highest processing areas" we mean areas responsible for multimodal association and integration, as well as high-level cognitive functions, like calculation, writing, thinking, drawing, problem-solving, conscious beliefs and desires, and not in the least highly complex mental processes, like creative artistic or scientific activities. Lower-level processing areas are responsible for less complex and more basic structures and functions of the nervous system, for instance, emotions (e.g., fear, panic, lust, joy, etc.) and the autonomic PNS components that I take as constitutive of these mental states (e.g., increased or decreased pulse and blood pressure, sweating, heat waves, trembling, etc.). Other such lower-level states are thirst, hunger, pain, touch, proprioception, and so on. We also, of course, include the somatic PNS, sensory and motor, in the category of lower-level processing areas, together with reflex behavior at that level.

It might not appear that it hits the nail on the head, but I think that the principle is plausible and offers intuitive answers in various cases. To start with the very last clause of PP, it sanctions as permissible cosmetic surgery, given that cosmetic surgery is understood in terms of intervention types that do not interfere with important functions of the organism. Correcting the shape of a nose or a breast does not interfere with the main functions of these organs. However, when the affected part of the nervous system is large enough or crucial for the right manifestation of a function of the organism, PP gives precedence to more basic processing and functional areas of the nervous system, so that their being kept intact is more important than the request of the patient, unless the neural basis of the need that would be satisfied by the intervention is at a more basic level than the level at which the intervention would be effected. Let us consider some examples.

First, consider an example when a patient has developed obsessive thoughts, worries, enforced by imaginative processes, about falling when going downstairs, because his legs are weak, so when he faces the situation of walking downstairs, his autonomic nervous system overreacts; he trembles and is unable to even move his lower limbs. His legs are not weak at all; they are completely normal, but his extreme nervousness when he faces the stairs blocks him. Suppose that medication did not work so far, so the patient requests surgery. There are, presumably, three main types of possible destructive surgery requests that would alleviate the condition: amputation of the lower limbs, disconnection of the amygdala from the autonomic nervous system (or destruction of a part of the amygdala), and disconnection or destruction of some higher cortical structures responsible for the maintenance of thoughts or imagination. The first option would alleviate the condition because the patient would use special, external aids for locomotion, involving his use of the upper limbs, whose function is not affected by this phobia. The second option would also alleviate the condition by emotionally desensitizing the patient when confronted with the relevant stimulus. The amygdala is responsible for fear conditioning and emotional memory, so destroying the relevant part of it would make the patient fearless when it comes to confronting the previously dreaded situation. Finally, making the relevant disconnection or destruction at the higher levels of processing would stop the escalation of thoughts and imagination, and would overcome obsession.

For all of these interventions, when we assert that they are permissible, we are implicitly assuming a ceteris paribus clause, so that we exclude other effects of the intervention than the desired result.

The PP principle would rule that it is not permissible to intervene on the legs as compared to a potential intervention on the amygdala or the higher cortical areas because the need is that of becoming free from obsessive thoughts, which is above the level of the legs. As regards the higher levels, it is then an open question, as far as PP is concerned, whether it is permissible to intervene upon them.

Next, consider a more intuitive case for PP, if the previous one does not immediately appear so. Suppose a painter suffers from major depression and that no medication has been effective in his case. Because of his depression he stops painting and develops negative thoughts to the effect that he is worthless. He is a fan of Vincent Van Gogh and has come to believe that he would be more creative if he imitated his idol and removed one of his ears, so he requests such an operation from a surgeon. PP will rule that if surgical intervention is the only viable option, it should not take place at the level of the ear, as the ear is at a much more basic level than the level at which the need is neurally realized. The need is realized at very high levels of processing, those that have to do with self-image, self-worth, perception of the other, and so on, which is probably the cingulate cortex.

The general point of PP is that basic, low-level, hard-wired parts of the nervous system have priority over complex, high-level, highly plastic parts. Going back to the problem of amputation, if any surgery is necessary to alleviate the BIID patients' suffering, it will have to take place at a certain level of the nervous system, according as where the need expressed by the desire to have one's limb amputated is situated. It is, of course, a matter of controversy at which level of the nervous system the real need ultimately is. However, even if Bayne and Levi are right that we could ascribe an illness to the limb, "or at least, the neuronal representation of it," there is a big difference, from the point of view of PP, between whether we ascribe to the limb or to its neuronal representation in the brain. If the patients' limbs don't appear to be dysfunctional, so that their body schema appears as unaffected, then, if any surgery is needed, it has to take place not at the level of the limbs, but at some level in the brain, where the neuronal representation of the limb is realized.

In any case, if BIID is ultimately a desire to be disabled, with a wide-ranging scale of particular types of disability (blindness, deafness, paralysis, amputation) as the newer definition suggests, then the need is likely to be a complex, high-level one, related to self-image and social interaction, and I then hardly see any reason for the requested surgery to be permissible. Instead, the recommendation would be to act on the relevant parts of the brain in order to change the peculiar beliefs that the patient has developed, if such an option is available at all. Some BIID patients insist on the parallel with sex change surgery and transgender people, but, as I have pointed out before, sex change operation does not merely destroy some organs, or replace them with ones that have the very same structure and function (as it happened in the case of a BIID patient presented in the documentary *Whole*, who shot himself in the leg, got as a result his leg amputated, and now wears a prosthetic leg). Moreover, arguably, these patients' request of sex change surgery is based on a need that is partly realized at the same level (i.e., genital organs) as the level at which the requested operation would take place. Hence, PP would rule that sex change surgery is permissible.

10

Concluding Remarks

I have tried in this book to offer a new approach to many extant problems in the philosophy of mind, based on taking the peripheral nervous system (PNS) seriously. Contemporary philosophy of mind has truly been fixated on the brain as the seat of mentality, and there has been an almost complete neglect of the conceptual role the PNS might play in solving many philosophical conundrums.

As I have also tried to show, even the newest and increasingly popular "embodied and embedded cognition" (EEC) literature sometimes fails to take the PNS as such seriously. EEC insists, of course, on a concept of mind and cognition that essentially involves the body and the environment, but, nevertheless, there is no explicit recognition of the PNS as being essential to mentality; presumably, it is taken on a par with how the brain is understood in cognitivism, the view that EEC is supposed to be an alternative to, or even worse, as an anatomical unit that apparently does not have any potential interesting philosophical import.

Similar observations apply to particular approaches within EEC, like the extended mind (EM) hypothesis and *Enactivism*. Neither of them focuses on the specific role the PNS plays in nervous systems and by extension in the concept of mind or particular mental phenomena. The EM hypothesis, just like other EEC approaches and like standard Putnam-style externalism, is interested in bringing the mind beyond the margins of the skull, deep into the world. Even though the EM hypothesis is presented as very different from classical semantic externalism in that it is an *active externalism*, they still share something important, namely, the belief that the mind extends not only beyond the brain but also beyond the nervous system. The *brain/nervous system distinction* is rarely made in the literature; that is why the champions of EM seem to implicitly think that because there are good reasons to believe that the mind is not confined to the brain, the mind must be taken as partly outside the nervous system and the body as a whole. Enactivism has a similar prejudice, and many more problems, which I have expounded in chapter 8 of this book.

To my knowledge, there is currently no extensive philosophical work that specifically discusses the PNS per se as part of a viable concept of the mind. On the contrary, classical, analytic philosophy type of works, many times based on poor empirical knowledge of the nervous system, are focused on "the brain," leaving the discussion at this overly general level. As mentioned above, even the EEC approach leaves the PNS underdiscussed, possibly because its supporters have thought that there cannot be anything more interesting about the PNS beyond the fact that it is an appendix to the central nervous system (CNS), therefore, if one cared about the PNS, one would still be working within the old cognitivist, brain and symbolic representation based paradigm.

I have tried to argue in this book that elegant solutions to philosophical problems are available once we augment our view of mental states with the hypothesis that the PNS is essential to or constitutive of them. The idea is far from being ad hoc. The neuroscience literature—theoretical, experimental, clinical, and therapeutic—is clear evidence against both classical philosophy of mind, which implicitly understands mental states as *terminus* points of causal chains that end in some area of the brain (usually assumed to be somewhere on the cortex), and against the newer, EEC type approaches, which many times go to the other extreme, of placing the mind beyond the body. A good example of such neuroscientific evidence was presented in chapters 3 and 4, where I have analyzed the conceptual relevance of the best neuroscientific theory of pain mechanisms, the Gate Control Theory of Pain (GCTP). As I have tried to show in those chapters, GCTP makes it clear that there is no such thing as a "pain center" in the brain, unless the whole brain is taken as a "center," and even under that assumption the idea of a pain center is meaningless. At the same time, the PNS could clearly and coherently be understood as having a constitutive role to the phenomenal state of pain.

There are several other philosophical problems that my approach has proved to address from a fresh perspective and has attempted to solve in an original way. The reader will ultimately judge whether these attempts were successful, but my main goal was to basically

reshuffle the deck of cards a bit in order to see the problems differently. Most of these solutions will be based on the correct neuroscience, which leads to what I put forward as the correct *folk
neuroscience* to be used in addressing philosophical issues about the
mind-body relation. Other solutions are based on first-person phenomenological reflection, so that my approach hopefully does not
fail to account for first-person data. In fact, the introductory chapter
to the book described my personal experiences related to severe
peripheral nerve damage of the motor nerves that I suffered in 2005,
due to chemotoxicity during chemotherapeutic treatment for Hodgkin's Lymphoma. As mentioned in that chapter, those experiences—
like proprioceptively feeling my feet as foreign bodies attached to
my "real feet," having to reinvent moving my arms and feet based
on visual data rather than on proprioceptive ones, the weirdness of
sensing any thermal, pain, and touch stimulus while failing to have
a motor response to it at the level of the limbs, and so on—made me
first think about the importance of the PNS for consciousness and
wonder whether the philosophy of mind has something interesting
to say about it. Over the last few years I had a few occasions to
reflect on this conjecture, and I have come to think that a reinterpretation of mental concepts in light of a constitutive role of the PNS
has a non-negligible potential to offer new insights into traditional
philosophical problems. I can only hope, in light of the numerous
fascinating works in this field that are being published every year,
that the results of these reflections, now embodied in this book, will
not end up being peripheral.

References

Adams, F., and K. Aizawa. 2001. "The Bounds of Cognition." *Philosophical Psychology* 14: 43–64.

———. 2008. "Why the Mind Is Still in the Head." Pp. 78–96 in *Cambridge Handbook on Situated Cognition*, ed. P. Robbins and Murat Aydede. New York: Cambridge University Press.

Appiah, K. A. 2004. "Akan and Euro-American Concepts of the Person." Pp. 21–34 in *African Philosophy*, ed. Lee Brown. New York: Oxford University Press.

———. 2008. *Experiments in Ethics*. Cambridge, MA: Harvard University Press.

Aranyosi, I. 2007. "Shadows of Constitution." *The Monist* 90 (3): 315–32.

———. 2010. "Powers and the Mind-Body Problem." *International Journal of Philosophical Studies* 18 (1): 57–72.

———. 2011. "A New Argument for Mind-Brain Identity." *British Journal for the Philosophy of Science* 62 (3): 489–517.

Arcaro, M. J., et al. 2011. "Visuotopic Organization of Macaque Posterior Parietal Cortex: A Functional Magnetic Resonance Imaging Study." *Journal of Neuroscience* 31 (6): 2064–78.

Armstrong, D. M. [1968] 2002. *A Materialist Theory of the Mind*. London and New York: Routledge.

Azmitia, E. C. 1999. "Serotonin Neurons, Neuroplasticity, and Homeostasis of Neural Tissue." *Neuropsychopharmacology* 21: 33S–45S.

———. 2007. "Cajal and Brain Plasticity: Insights Relevant to Emerging Concepts of Mind." *Brain Research Review* 55: 395–405.

Balog, K. 1999. "Conceivability, Possibility, and the Mind–Body Problem." *Philosophical Review* 108: 497–528.

———. 2009. "Phenomenal Concepts." Pp. 292–312 in *Oxford Handbook in the Philosophy of Mind*, ed. Brian McLaughlin, Ansgar Beckermann, and Sven Walter. New York: Oxford University Press.

———. 2012. "In Defense of the Phenomenal Concept Strategy." *Philosophy and Phenomenological Research* 84 (1): 1–23.

Batty, C. 2010. "A Representational Account of Olfactory Experience." *Canadian Journal of Philosophy* 40 (4): 511–38.

Bayne, T., and N. Levy. 2005. "Amputees by Choice: Body Integrity Identity Disorder and the Ethics of Amputation." *Journal of Applied Philosophy* 22 (1): 75–86.

Bechtel, W., and A. Abrahamsen. 1991. *Connectionism and the Mind: An Introduction to Parallel Processing in Networks*. Cambridge, MA: Basil Blackwell.

Beer, R. D. 2000. "Dynamical Approaches to Cognitive Science." *Trends in Cognitive Science* 4: 91–99.

———. forthcoming. "Dynamical Systems and Embedded Cognition." In *The Cambridge Handbook of Artificial Intelligence*, ed. K. Frankish and W. Ramsey. Cambridge: Cambridge University Press.

Benedetti, F. 1985. "Processing of Tactile Spatial Information with Crossed Fingers." *Journal of Experimental Psychology* 11 (4): 517–25.

———. 1986. "Tactile Diplopia (Diplesthesia) on the Human Fingers." *Perception* 15 (1): 83–91.

———. 1990. "Goal Directed Motor Behavior and Its Adaptation Following Reversed Tactile Perception in Man." *Experimental Brain Research* 81 (1): 70–76.

———. 1991. "Perceptual Learning following a Long Lasting Tactile Reversal." *Journal of Experimental Psychology* 17 (1): 267–77.

Bensler, M. J., and D. S. Paauw. 2003. "Apotemnophilia Masquerading as Medical Morbidity." *Southern Medical Journal* 96 (7): 674–76.

Berger, P. L., and T. Luckmann. 1966. *The Social Construction of Reality: A Treatise in the Sociology of Knowledge*. Garden City, NY: Anchor Books.

Berlucchi, G., and S. M. Aglioti. 2010. "The Body in the Brain Revisited." *Experimental Brain Research* 200: 25–35.

Bermúdez, J. L. 1998. *The Paradox of Self-Consciousness*. Cambridge, MA: MIT Press.

Birt, R. E. 1991. "Review: Identity and the Question of African Philosophy." *Philosophy East and West* 41 (1): 95–109.

Blakemore, C. 2006. "Preface." Pp. v–vi in *Neuroethics*, ed. J. Illes. New York: Oxford University Press.

Block, N. [1978] 2002. "Troubles with Functionalism." Pp. 94–98 in *Philosophy of Mind: Classical and Contemporary Readings*, ed. D. J. Chalmers. New York: Oxford University Press.

———. 2005. "Review of Alva Noë." *Journal of Philosophy* 102: 259–72.

Blumberg, M. S. 2010. "Beyond Dreams: Do Sleep-Related Movements Contribute to Brain Development?" *Frontiers in Neurology* 1: 140.

Botvinick, M., and J. Cohen. 1998. "Rubber Hands 'Feel' Touch that Eyes See." *Nature* 391: 756.

Bridy, A. 2004. "Confounding Extremities: Surgery at the Medicoethical Limits of Self-modification." *Journal of Law, Medicine and Ethics* 32 (1): 148–58.

Bullier, J. 2001. "Integrated Model of Visual Processing." *Brain Research Reviews* 36: 96–107.

Burge, T. 1979. "Individualism and the Mental." *Midwest Studies in Philosophy* 4: 73–121.

Cage, J. [1939] 1961. *Silence*, Middletown, CT: Wesleyan University Press.

Cahan, D., ed. 1993. *Hermann von Helmoltz and the Foundations of Nineteenth-Century Science*. Berkeley and Los Angeles: University of California Press.

Carlstedt, Th., et al. 2004. "Spinal Cord in Relation to Peripheral Nervous System." Pp. 250–66 in *The Human Nervous System*, ed. G. Paxinos and Jürgen K. Mai. San Diego, CA: Elsevier Academic Press.

Chalmers, D. J. 1996. *The Conscious Mind: In Search of a Fundamental Theory*. New York: Oxford University Press.

———. 2005. "The Matrix as Metaphysics." Pp. 132–176 in *Philosophers Explore the Matrix*, ed. C. Grau. New York: Oxford University Press.

Chevillet, M., et al. 2011. "Functional Correlates of the Anterolateral Processing Hierarchy in Human Auditory Cortex." *Journal of Neuroscience* 31 (25): 9345–9352.

Churchland, P. S. 2006. "Moral Decision-Making and the Brain." Pp. 3–16 in *Neuroethics*, ed. J. Illes. New York: Oxford University Press.

Clark, A. 2008. *Supersizing the Mind*. New York: Oxford University Press.

———. 2009. "Spreading the Joy? Why the Machinery of Consciousness is (Probably) Still in the Head." *Mind* 118 (472): 963–93.

———. 2010. "*Memento*'s Revenge: The Extended Mind, Extended." Pp. 43–67 in *The Extended Mind*, ed. R. Menary. Cambridge, MA: MIT Press.

Clark, A., and D. Chalmers. 1998. "The Extended Mind." *Analysis* 58: 10–23.

Clarke, C. J. S. 1995. "The Nonlocality of Mind." *Journal of Consciousness Studies* 2 (3): 231–40.

Conee, E. 1999. "Metaphysics and the Morality of Abortion." *Mind* 108 (432): 619–45.

Cowey, A. 2005. "The Ferrier Lecture 2004: What can Transcranial Magnetic Stimulation Tell Us about How the Brain Works?" *Philosophical Transactions of the Royal Society B* 360: 1185–1205.

Craig, A. D. 2003. "Interoception: The Sense of the Physiological Condition of the Body." *Current Opinion in Neurobiology* 13: 500–505.

Crane, T. 1991. "All the Difference in the World." *Philosophical Quarterly* 41: 1–25.

Crerand, C. E., et al. 2006. "Body Dysmorphic Disorder and Cosmetic Surgery." *Plastic and Reconstructive Surgery* 118 (7): 167e–80e.

Crick, F., and Ch. Koch. 1995. "Are We Aware of Neural Activity in Primary Visual Cortex?" *Nature* 375: 121–23.

Csíkszentmihályi, M. 1990. *Flow: The Psychology of Optimal Experience.* New York: Harper and Row.

Dacey, D. M., and B. B. Lee. 1994. "The 'Blue-On' Opponent Pathway in Primate Retina Originates from a Distinct Bistratified Ganglion Cell Type." *Nature* 367: 731–35.

Dalton, T. C., and V. W. Bergenn. 2007. *Early Experience, the Brain, and Consciousness: An Historical and Interdisciplinary Synthesis.* New York: Taylor and Francis.

Damasio, A. R. 1994. *Descartes' Error: Emotion, Reason, and the Human Brain.* New York: Putnam Publishing.

———. 2003. *Looking for Spinoza: Joy, Sorrow, and the Feeling Brain.* New York: Harcourt.

———. 2010. *Self Comes to Mind: Constructing the Conscious Brain.* New York: Pantheon Books.

Damasio, A. R., et al. 1990. "Individuals with Sociopathic Behavior Caused by Frontal Damage Fail to Respond Autonomically to Social Stimuli." *Behavior and Brain Research* 41: 81–94.

Decosterd, I., and C. J. Woolf. 2000. "Spared Nerve Injury: An Animal Model of Persistent Peripheral Neuropathic Pain." *Pain* 87 (2): 149–58.

Dennett, D. C. 1991. *Consciousness Explained.* Boston, New York, London: Little, Brown and Company.

———. 2000. "Making Tools for Thinking." Pp. 17–29 in *Metarepresentations: A Multidisciplinary Perspective,* ed. D. Sperber. Oxford: Oxford University Press.

Diaz-Leon, E. 2008. "Defending the Phenomenal Concept Strategy." *Australasian Journal of Philosophy* 86 (4): 597–610.

———. 2010. "Can Phenomenal Concepts Explain the Epistemic Gap?" *Mind* 119 (476): 933–51.

Dyl, J., Kittler, J., et al. 2006. "Body Dysmorphic Disorder and Other Clinically Significant Body Image Concerns in Adolescent Psychiatric Inpatients: Prevalence and Clinical Characteristics." *Child Psychiatry and Human Development* 36: 369–82.

Ehrsson, H. H. 2009. "How Many Arms Make a Pair? Perceptual Illusion of Having an Additional Limb." *Perception* 38: 310–12.

Elliott, C. 2003. *Better than Well: American Medicine Meets the American Dream.* New York: W. W. Norton and Co.

Fabian, J. [1983] 2002. *Time and the Other: How Anthropology Makes Its Object.* New York: Columbia University Press.

Farkas, K. 2003. "What is Externalism?" *Philosophical Studies* 112 (3): 187–208.

Feenstra, M. G. P., and G. van der Plasse. 2010. "Tryptophan Depletion and Serotonin Release—A Critical Reappraisal." Pp. 249–58 in *Handbook of the Behavioral Neurobiology of Serotonin*, ed. C. P. Müller and B. L. Jacobs. London: Elsevier BV.

Feigl, H. 1958. "The 'Mental' and the 'Physical.'" Pp. 370–497 in *Concepts, Theories and the Mind-Body Problem*, ed. H. Feigl, M. Scriven, and G. Maxwell. Minnesota Studies in the Philosophy of Science, Vol. 2. Minneapolis.

First, M. B. 2004. "Desire for Amputation of a Limb: Paraphilia, Psychosis, or a New Type of Identity Disorder." *Psychological Medicine* 34: 1–10.

First, M. B., and C. E. Fisher 2012. "Body Integrity Identity Disorder: The Persistent Desire to Acquire a Physical Disability." *Psychopathology* 45: 3–14.

Fitzgerald, M. 2010. "The Lost Domain of Pain." *Brain* 133 (6): 1850–54.

Flower, M. J. 1985. "Neuromaturation of the Human Fetus." *Journal of Medicine and Philosophy* 10: 237–51.

Gallagher, S. 2003. "Bodily Self-Awareness and Object-Perception." *Theoria et Historia Scientiarum: International Journal for Interdisciplinary Studies* 7 (1): 53–68.

———. 2005. *How the Body Shapes the Mind*. New York: Oxford University Press.

———. 2012. "The Body in Social Context: Some Qualifications on the 'Warmth and Intimacy' of Bodily Self-consciousness." *Grazer Philosophische Studien* 84: 103–33.

Gallagher, S., and J. Cole. 1995. "Body Schema and Body Image in a Deafferented Subject." *Journal of Mind and Behavior* 16 (4): 369–90.

Gallup, G. G. Jr. 1970. "Chimpanzees: Self Recognition." *Science* 167 (3914): 86–87.

Garcia-Segura, L. M. 2009. *Hormones and Brain Plasticity*. New York: Oxford University Press.

Gazzaniga, M. 2005. *The Ethical Brain*. New York: Dana Press.

———. 2006. "Facts, Fictions, and the Future of Neuroethics." Pp. 141–48 in *Neuroethics: Defining the Issues in Theory, Practice, and Policy*, ed. J. Illes. New York: Oxford University Press.

Gibson, J. J. 1966. *The Senses Considered as Perceptual Systems*. Boston: Houghton Mifflin.

———. 1979. *The Ecological Approach to Visual Perception*. Boston: Houghton Mifflin.

Godfrey-Smith, P. 2009. "Triviality Arguments against Functionalism." *Philosophical Studies* 145: 273–95.

Goebel, R., et al. 2001. "Sustained Extrastriate Cortical Activation without Visual Awareness Revealed by fMRI Studies of Hemianopic Patients." *Vision Research* 41: 1459–74.

Goebel, R., L. Muckli, and D.-S. Kim. 2004. "Visual System." Pp. 1280–306 in *The Human Nervous System*, ed. G. Paxinos and Jürgen K. Mai. San Diego, CA: Elsevier, Inc.

Gyekye, K. [1987] 1995. *The Akan Conceptual Scheme: An Essay on African Philosophical Thought*, revised edition. Philadelphia: Temple University Press.

Haller, J., et al. 1998. "Catecholaminergic Involvement in the Control of Aggression: Hormones, the Peripheral Sympathetic, and Central Noradrenergic Systems." *Neuroscience and Biobehavioral Reviews* 22 (1): 85–97.

Harris, C. S. 1963. "Adaptation to Displaced Vision: Visual, Motor, or Proprioceptive Change?" *Science* 140 (3568): 812–13.

———. 1965. "Perceptual Adaptation to Inverted, Reversed, and Displaced Vision." *Psychological Review* 72 (6): 419–44.

Hart, W. D. 1988. *The Engines of the Soul*. Cambridge: Cambridge University Press.

Heil, J. 1989. "Recent Work in Realism and Anti-Realism." *Philosophical Books* 30 (2): 65–73.

Held, R. 1961. "Exposure-History as a Factor in Maintaining Stability of Perception and Coordination." *Journal of Nervous and Mental Disease* 132: 26–32.

Held, R., and J. Bossom 1961. "Neonatal Deprivation and Adult Rearrangement: Complementary Techniques for Analyzing Plastic Sensory-Motor Coordinations." *Journal of Comparative and Physiological Psychology* 54: 33–37.

Held, R., and S. J. Freedman. 1963. "Plasticity in Human Sensorimotor Control." *Science* 142: 455–62.

Held, R., and A. Hein. 1963. "Movement Produced Stimulation in the Development of Visually Guided Behavior." *Journal of Comparative and Physiological Psychology* 56: 873–76.

Held, R., and J. Rekosh. 1963. "Motor-Sensory Feedback and the Geometry of Visual Space." *Science* 141: 722–23.

Horgan, T., and J. Tienson. 2002. "The Intentionality of Phenomenology and the Phenomenology of Intentionality." Pp. 520–33 in *Philosophy of Mind: Classical and Contemporary Readings*, ed. D. J. Chalmers. Oxford and New York: Oxford University Press.

Hurley, S. 1998. *Consciousness in Action*. Cambridge, MA: Harvard University Press.

Hurley, S., and A. Noë. 2003. "Neural Plasticity and Consciousness." *Biology and Philosophy* 18 (1): 131–68.

Husserl, E. [1913] 1962. *Ideas: General Introduction to Pure Phenomenology* (also known as Ideas I). Trans. W. Boyce Gibson. New York: Collier Books.

Illes, J., ed. 2006. *Neuroethics: Defining the Issues in Theory, Practice, and Policy*. New York: Oxford University Press.

Jackson, F. C. 1982. "Epiphenomenal Qualia." *Philosophical Quarterly* 32: 127–36.

———. 1998. "Reference and Description Revisited." *Philosophical Perspectives* 12: 201–18.

Jaynes, J. [1976] 2000. *The Origin of Consciousness in the Breakdown of the Bicameral Mind*. New York: Mariner Books.

Johnson, S. C., et al. 2002. "Neural Correlates of Self-Reflection." *Brain* 125 (8): 1808–14.

Kamm, F. M. 1992. *Creation and Abortion: A Study in Moral and Legal Philosophy*. New York: Oxford University Press.

Kar, K., and B. Krekelberg. 2012. "Transcranial Electrical Stimulation over Visual Cortex Evokes Phosphenes with a Retinal Origin." *Journal of Neurophysiology* 108 (8): 2173–78.

Klein, C. 2007. "Kicking the Kohler Habit." *Philosophical Psychology* 20 (5): 609–19.

Kohler, I. 1961. "Experiments with Goggles." *Scientific American* 206: 62–72.

———. 1964. "The Formation and Transformation of the Perceptual World." *Psychological Issues* 3: 1–173.

Kripke, S. [1972] 2006. *Naming and Necessity*. Malden, MA: Blackwell Publishing.

Kroon, F. 1987. "Causal Descriptivism." *Australasian Journal of Philosophy* 65: 1–17.

Lagercrantz, H., and J.-P. Changeux. 2009. "The Emergence of Human Consciousness: From Fetal to Neonatal Life." *Pediatric Research* 65 (3): 255–60.

Lakoff, G., and M. Johnson. 1999. *Philosophy in the Flesh: The Embodied Mind and its Challenge to Western Thought*. New York: Basic Books.

Lamme, V. A., and P. R. Roelfsema. 2000. "The Distinct Modes of Vision Offered by Feedforward and Recurrent Processing." *Trends in Neuroscience* 23: 571–79.

Lee, S. J. et al. 2005. "Fetal Pain: A Systematic Multidisciplinary Review of the Evidence." *Journal of the American Medical Association* 294 (8): 947–54.

Lewis, D. K. 1966. "An Argument for the Identity Theory." *Journal of Philosophy* 63: 17–25.

———. 1980. "Mad Pain and Martian Pain." Pp. 102–15 in *Problems in Mind: Readings in Contemporary Philosophy of Mind*, ed. J. S. Crumley II. Mountain View, CA: Mayfield Publishing Company, 2000.

———. 1984. "Putnam's Paradox." *Australasian Journal of Philosophy* 62: 221–36.

———. [1988] 2004. "What Experience Teaches." Pp. 75–104 in *There is Something about Mary*, ed. P. Ludlow, Y. Nagasawa, and D. Stoljar. Cambridge, MA: MIT Press.

Linden, D. E., et al. 1999. "The Myth of Upright Vision: A Psychophysical and Functional Imaging Study of Adaptation to Inverting Spectacles." *Perception* 28: 469–81.

Loar, B. [1990] 1997. "Phenomenal States" (Revised Version). Pp. 597–616 in *The Nature of Consciousness: Philosophical Debates*, ed. N. Block, O. Flanagan, G. Güzeldere. Cambridge, MA: MIT Press.

Lycan, W. 2000. "The Slighting of Smell." Pp. 273–90 in *Of Minds and Molecules: New Philosophical Perspectives on Chemistry*, ed. N. Bhushan and S. Rosenfeld. New York: Oxford University Press.

Mallon, R., E. Machery, S. Nichols, and S. Stich. 2004. "Semantics Cross-Cultural Style." *Cognition* 92: B1–B12.

Marr, D. [1982] 2010. *Vision*. Cambridge, MA: MIT Press.

Mellor, D. H. 1977. "Natural Kinds." *British Journal for the Philosophy of Science* 28 (4): 299–312.

Melzack, R., and P. D. Wall. 1965. "Pain Mechanisms: A New Theory." *Science* 150 (3699): 971–79.

Menary, R. 2007. *Cognitive Integration: Mind and Cognition Unbounded*. Houndmills, UK: Palgrave Macmillan.

———. 2010. "Cognitive Integration and the Extended Mind." Pp. 227–44 in *The Extended Mind*, ed. R. Menary. Cambridge, MA: MIT Press.

Merker, B. 2007. "Consciousness without a Cerebral Cortex: A Challenge for Neuroscience and Medicine." *Behavioral and Brain Sciences* 30: 63–134.

Merleau-Ponty, M. [1945] 2002. *Phenomenology of Perception*. London: Routledge.

———. [1995] 2003. *Nature: Course Notes from the College de France*. Ed. D. Seglard and trans. R. Vallier. Evanston, IL: Northwestern University Press.

Miller, N. M., et al. 2005. "The Fetal Patient." Pp. 1–16 in *Anesthesia for Fetal Intervention and Surgery*, ed. L. B. Myers and L. A. Bulich. Hamilton, Ontario: BC Decker Inc.

Millikan, R. G.. 1993. "What is Behavior?" Pp. 135–50 in *White Queen Psychology and Other Essays for Alice*, ed. R. G. Millikan. Cambridge, MA: MIT Press.

Mombaerts, P., et al. 1996. "Visualizing an Olfactory Sensory Map." *Cell* 87 (4): 675–86.

Myin, E., and J. O'Regan. 2009. "Situated Perception and Sensation in Vision and Other Modalities: A Sensorimotor Approach." Pp. 185–200 in *Cambridge Handbook of Situated Cognition*, ed. P. Robbins and M. Aydede. Cambridge: Cambridge University Press.

Nagel, T. 1974. "What Is It Like to be a Bat?" *Philosophical Review* 4: 435–50.

Nida-Rümelin, M. [1996] 2002. "Pseudonormal Vision: A Case of Actual Qualia Inversion?" Pp. 99–105 in *Philosophy of Mind: Classical and Contemporary Readings*, ed. D. J. Chalmers. New York: Oxford University Press.

Noë, A. 2004. *Action in Perception*. Cambridge, MA: MIT Press.

O'Regan, J., and A. Noë. 2001. "A Sensorimotor Account of Vision and Visual Consciousness." *Behavioral and Brain Sciences* 24: 939–1031.

O'Shaughnessy, B. 1995. "Proprioception and the Body Image." Pp. 175–203 in *The Body and the Self*, ed. J. L. Bermúdez, A. J. Marcel, and N. Eilan. Cambridge, MA: MIT Press.

———. 2000. *Consciousness and the World*. Oxford: Oxford University Press.

Papineau, D. 2002. *Thinking about Consciousness*. New York: Oxford University Press.

———. 2007. "Phenomenal and Perceptual Concepts." Pp. 111–44 in *Phenomenal Concepts and Phenomenal Knowledge: New Essays on Consciousness and Physicalism*, ed. Torin Alter and Sven Walter. New York: Oxford University Press.

Parsons, J. 2004. "Distributional Properties." Pp. 173–80 in *Lewisian Themes: The Philosophy of David K. Lewis*, ed. Frank Jackson and Graham Priest. Oxford: Oxford University Press.

Paxinos, G., and Jürgen K. Mai, eds. 2004. *The Human Nervous System*. San Diego, CA: Elsevier Academic Press

Peacocke, Ch. 1983. *Sense and Content: Experience, Thought and their Relations*. New York: Oxford University Press.

Perry, M. C., and N. F. McKinney. 2008. "Chemotherapeutic Agents." Pp. 575–633 in *The Chemotherapy Sourcebook*, Fourth edition, ed. M. C. Perry. Philadelphia, PA: Lippincott Williams and Wilkins.

Place, U. T. 1956. "Is Consciousness a Brain Process?" *British Journal of Psychology* 47 (1): 44–50.

Plotnik, J. M., et al. 2006. "Self-recognition in an Asian Elephant." *Proceedings of the National Academy of Sciences USA* 103: 17053–57.

Prinz, J. 2006. "Putting the Brakes on Enactive Perception." *Psyche* 12 (1): 1–19.

Puccetti, R. 1977. "The Great C-Fiber Myth." *Philosophy of Science* 44: 303–5.

Putnam, H. 1973. "Meaning and Reference." *Journal of Philosophy* 70 (19): 699–711.

———. 1975. "The Meaning of 'Meaning'." *Minnesota Studies in the Philosophy of Science* 7: 131–93.

———. 1982. *Reason, Truth and History*. Cambridge: Cambridge University Press.

———. 1990. *Realism with a Human Face*. Cambridge, MA: Harvard University Press.

Ralston, H. J. 1984. "Synaptic Organization of Spinothalamic Tract Projections to the Thalamus, with Special Reference to Pain." Pp. 183–95 in *Advances in Pain Research and Therapy*, ed. L. Kruger and J. C. Liebeskind. New York: Raven Press.

Ramachandran, V. S., and W. Hirstein. 1998. "The Perception of Phantom Limbs. The D. O. Hebb Lecture." *Brain* 121: 1603–30.

Rees, G., G. Kreiman, and C. Koch. 2002. "Neural Correlates of Consciousness in Humans." *Nature Reviews Neuroscience* 3: 261–70.

Rees, S., and D. Walker. 2001. "Nervous and Neuromuscular Systems." Pp. 154–85 in *Fetal Growth and Development*, ed. R. Harding and A. D. Bocking. Cambridge: Cambridge University Press.

Reiss, D., and L. Marino. 2001. "Mirror Self-Recognition in the Bottlenose Dolphin: A Case of Cognitive Convergence." *Proceedings of the National Academy of Sciences USA* 98: 5937–42.

Rivers, W. H. R. 1894. "A Modification of Aristotle's Experiment." *Mind* 3 (12): 583–84.

Robertson, G. C. 1876. "Sense of Doubleness with Crossed Fingers." *Mind* 1 (1): 145–46.

Roorda, A., and D. R. Williams. 1999. "The Arrangement of the Three Cone Classes in the Living Human Eye." *Nature* 397: 520–22.

Roskies, A. 2002. "Neuroethics for the New Millenium." *Neuron* 35: 21–23.

Rösler, A., and E. Witztum. 2000. "Pharmacotherapy of Paraphilias in the Next Millennium." *Behavioral Sciences and the Law* 18: 43–56.

Rowlands, M. 2010. *The New Science of the Mind: From Extended Mind to Embodied Phenomenology*. Cambridge, MA: MIT Press.

Rozin, P. 1982. "'Taste-Smell Confusions' and the Duality of the Olfactory Sense." *Perception and Psychophysics* 31 (4): 397–401.

Rumelhart, D. E., J. L. McClelland, and the PDP Research Group. 1986. *Parallel Distributed Processing: Explorations in the Microstructure of Cognition*. Volumes 1 and 2. Cambridge, MA: MIT Press.

Russo, S., et al. 2003. "Tryptophan as a Link between Psychopathology and Somatic States." *Psychosomatic Medicine* 65: 665–71.

Sartre, J.-P. [1956] 2011. *Being and Nothingness: A Phenomenological Essay in Ontology*. New York: Citadel Press.

Schellenberg, S. 2010. "Perceptual Experience and the Capacity to Act." Pp. 145–60 in *Perception, Action, and Consciousness*, ed. N. Gangopadhay, M. Madary, and F. Spicer. New York: Oxford University Press.

Schindler, H. J., et al. 1998. "Feedback Control during Mastication of Solid Food Textures—A Clinical-Experimental Study." *Journal of Prosthetic Dentistry* 80 (3): 330–36.

Schroer, R. 2010. "Where's the Beef? Phenomenal Concepts as Both Demonstrative and Substantial." *Australasian Journal of Philosophy* 88 (3): 505–22.

Schutter, D. J., and R. Hortensius. 2010. "Retinal Origin of Phosphenes to Transcranial Alternating Current Stimulation." *Clinical Neurophysiology* 121 (7): 1080–84.

Searle, J. 1983. *Intentionality: An Essay in the Philosophy of Mind*. Cambridge: Cambridge University Press.

Sebeok, Th. 2001. *Global Semiotics*. Bloomington: Indiana University Press.

Sereno, M. I., et al. 2001. "Mapping of Contralateral Space in Retinotopic Coordinates by a Parietal Cortical Area in Humans." *Science* 294 (5545): 1350–54.

Shapiro, L. 2010. *Embodied Cognition*. London and New York: Routledge.

Sill, E. R. [1900] 2001. "The Felt Location of the 'I'." Pp. 254–56 in *The Prose of Edward Rowland Sill*, ed. B. Rogers. New York: Elibron Classics.

Singer, P. 1993. *Practical Ethics*. Cambridge: Cambridge University Press.

———. 1996. *Rethinking Life and Death: The Collapse of Our Traditional Ethics*. New York: St. Martin's Griffin.

Smart, J. J. C. 1959. "Sensations and Brain Processes." *Philosophical Review* 68 (2): 141–56.

Smolensky, P. 1988. "On the Proper Treatment of Connectionism." *Behavioral and Brain Sciences* 11 (1): 1–23.

Stinneford, J. F. 2005. "Incapacitation Through Maiming: Chemical Castration, the Eighth Amendment, and the Denial of Human Dignity." *University of St. Thomas Law Journal* 3 (3): 559–688.

Stoljar, D. 2005. "Physicalism and Phenomenal Concepts." *Mind and Language* 20 (2): 296–302.

Stratton, G. 1897. "Vision without Inversion of the Retinal Image." *Psychological Review* 4: 341–60 and 463–81.

Sutton, J. 2010. "Exograms and Interdisciplinarity: History, the Extended Mind, and the Civilizing Process." Pp. 189–226 in *The Extended Mind*, ed. R. Menary. Cambridge, MA: MIT Press, 2010.

Taylor, J. G. 1963. *The Behavioral Basis of Perception*. New Haven: Yale University Press.

Telaranta, T. 2003. "Psychoneurological Applications of Endoscopic Sympathetic Blocks (ESB)." *Clinical Autonomic Research* 13 (1): 120–21.

Thelen, E., and L. B. Smith. 1994. *A Dynamic Systems Approach to the Development of Cognition and Action*. Cambridge, MA: MIT Press.

Thompson, E. 2007. *Mind and Life*. Cambridge, MA: Harvard University Press.

Thomson, J. J. 1971. "A Defense of Abortion." *Philosophy and Public Affairs* 1 (1): 47–66.

Tomasini, F. 2006. "Exploring Ethical Justification for Self-Demand Amputation." *Ethics and Medicine* 22 (2): 99–115.

Tong, F. 2003. "Primary Visual Cortex and Visual Awareness." *Nature Reviews Neuroscience* 4: 219–29.

Tooley, M. 1972. "Abortion and Infanticide." *Philosophy and Public Affairs* 2 (1): 37–65.

———. 1984. *Abortion and Infanticide*. New York: Oxford University Press.

Tye, M. 1995. "A Representational Theory of Pains and their Phenomenal Character." *Philosophical Perspectives* 9: 223–39.

———. 1999. "Phenomenal Consciousness: The Explanatory Gap as a Cognitive Illusion." *Mind* 108 (432): 705–25.

Van Essen, D. C., and J. H. R. Maunsell. 1983. "Hierarchical Organization and Functional Streams in the Visual Cortex." *Trends in Neuroscience* 6: 370–75.

Van Gelder, T. 1995. "What Might Cognition Be If Not Computation?" *Journal of Philosophy* 91: 345–81.

———. 1998. "The Dynamical Hypothesis Is Cognitive Science." *Behavioral and Brain Sciences* 21: 615–28.

Varela, F., E. Thompson, and E. Rosch 1991. *The Embodied Mind: Cognitive Science and Human Experience*. Cambridge, MA: MIT Press.

von Uexküll, J. [1934] 2010. *A Foray into the Worlds of Animals and Humans, with a Theory of Meaning*. Trans. Joseph D. O'Neil. Minneapolis: University of Minnesota Press.

Williamson, T. 2000. *Knowledge and Its Limits*. Oxford: Oxford University Press.

———. 2007. *The Philosophy of Philosophy*. Oxford: Wiley-Blackwell.

Yerramilli, D., and S. Johnsen. 2010. "Spatial Vision in the Purple Sea Urchin, *Strongylocentrotus purpuratus* (Echinoidea)." *Journal of Experimental Biology* 213: 249–55.

Zemach, E. M. 1976. "Putnam's Theory on the Reference of Substance Terms." *Journal of Philosophy* 73 (15): 116–27.

Name Index

221

Subject Index